The Transradial Handbook

Access site techniques for invasive cardiology and interventional radiology procedures have undergone rapidly evolving technological advances, with radial access offering important benefits for patients and health-care systems. This book provides a concise practical guide to the practice of transradial procedures in both specialties. It is a readily accessible source of information that provides evidence-based guidelines from extensive global literature, interpreted and contextualised by experienced and recognised international opinion leaders. It provides an overview of relevant trial data, cannulation technique, catheter selection and manipulation, catheter delivery, right heart catheterisation, and complication management. It offers a comprehensive but portable reference to aid learning for cardiology and radiology professionals and trainees.

Key Features:

- Fills a current gap in a growing transradial market with a contemporary approach.
- Guides cardiology and radiology practitioners and other health-care professionals in optimal performance of transradial access procedures.
- Draws from the experience of world experts, providing a ready reference pocketbook for easy access.

The Transradial Handbook
Evidence-based Practice

Edited by

James Nolan, MBChB, MD, FRCP
Professor of Cardiology
Keele University
Staffordshire, United Kingdom

Associate Editors

Thomas Johnson, BSc, MBBS, MD
Professor of Cardiology
Royal Infirmary
Bristol, United Kingdom

Karim Ratib, MBChB, MRCP
Consultant Structural and Interventional Cardiologist
University Hospital of North Midlands
Staffordshire, United Kingdom

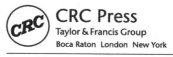

CRC Press
Taylor & Francis Group
Boca Raton London New York

CRC Press is an imprint of the
Taylor & Francis Group, an **informa** business

Designed cover image: cover image provided by James Nolan and Karim Ratib

First edition published 2025
by CRC Press
2385 NW Executive Center Drive, Suite 320, Boca Raton FL 33431

and by CRC Press
4 Park Square, Milton Park, Abingdon, Oxon, OX14 4RN

CRC Press is an imprint of Taylor & Francis Group, LLC

© 2025 selection and editorial matter, James Nolan individual chapters, the contributors

ISBN: 978-0-367-72142-8 (hbk)
ISBN: 978-0-367-72141-1 (pbk)
ISBN: 978-1-003-15362-7 (ebk)

DOI: 10.1201/9781003153627

Typeset in Times
by SPi Technologies India Pvt Ltd (Straive)

Contents

Preface

As an interventional trainee at the inception of the coronary stent era, I saw many severe access site complications. At this time, cardiology practice was to implant stents via large-diameter guiding catheters inserted into the femoral artery with accompanying heavy anticoagulation. The impact on patients who developed femoral access complications was severe. I was fortunate to attend one of the first transradial training courses at the OLVG hospital in Amsterdam – it was astonishing to see what could be achieved by switching from femoral to radial access. Returning to the OLVG as a transradial fellow the following year provided me with an incredible opportunity to develop my own transradial skills, which were invaluable in establishing a clinical and academic transradial programme in the United Kingdom (UK). Over time, cardiology practice in the UK evolved to become predominantly transradial, achieving major benefits for our patients. Cardiologists in the UK have made many contributions to the access site literature, helping to optimise and establish the technique internationally. A similar process of practice evolution is now underway in interventional radiology, albeit with technical challenges that are unique to the specialty. In this handbook, we have sought to provide easy-to-follow, evidence-based guidance to help operators at all levels of experience perform optimised transradial procedures and to deal with technical challenges and complications in both cardiology and interventional radiology. The goal of performing interventional procedures is to improve the health and quality of life of our patients, and the implementation of a transradial access programme is a significant means of limiting complications, improving quality of life, and achieving that objective.

James Nolan

The Editors

James Nolan, MBChB, MD, FRCP is Professor of Cardiology at Keele University in the UK. He trained in academic and interventional cardiology in London, Edinburgh, Leeds, and Amsterdam before taking up a National Health Service (NHS) consultant post at the University Hospital of North Midlands, where he established a large-scale programme of transradial cardiac procedures.

His areas of clinical practice relate to complex coronary intervention and percutaneous treatment of structural heart disease. The transradial programme at UHNM established it as a globally recognised centre of excellence for access site practice. He was a council member of the British Cardiovascular Intervention Society, setting up the society's international fellowship programme and its education and training group, and was a member of the national cardiology specialty advisory committee. He was actively involved in editorial roles with several journals and online educational forums and has made multiple contributions to international educational initiatives.

He led an active programme of education and training in optimised access site practice, running an annual transradial masterclass, as well as an international centre of excellence programme. His research interests cover all aspects of cardiovascular disease with a particular focus on the impact of radial access on outcomes of cardiac interventions. He has contributed to over 220 highly cited peer-reviewed publications, international guidelines on optimised radial practice, and more than 20 cardiology textbooks. This body of academic and educational activity has had significant practice changing impact on vascular access site practice and led to two lifetime achievement awards from national and international societies.

Thomas Johnson, BSc, MBBS, MD, FRCP is Associate Professor of Cardiology at the University of Bristol in the UK. He trained in academic and interventional cardiology in London, Bristol, and Auckland, New Zealand, before taking up an NHS consultant post at the Bristol Heart Institute at University Hospitals Bristol and Weston NHS Trust.

His areas of clinical practice relate to complex coronary intervention, with a particular focus on intracoronary imaging and bifurcation disease treatment. He led the development of the European Association of Percutaneous Coronary

Intervention consensus documents on the use of intracoronary imaging and is an active board member of the European Bifurcation Club, engaged in the regular publication of guidance for the interventional community. He has contributed to over 120 highly cited peer-reviewed publications and is a reviewer for multiple journals. As a UK interventionist, and through collaboration with Professor Nolan, he and his colleagues have developed a successful transradial programme in Bristol and educate and promote the benefits provided to patients and institutions through enhanced safety and improved efficiency.

As a board member of EuroPCR, he has been involved in the development of numerous educational initiatives spanning all levels of interventional experience. Through the use of simulation-based learning, he is directing a number of courses for fellows and interventional colleagues to accelerate their learning from vascular access to decision-making in PCI and the management of complications. His academic work spans discovery science, translation into clinic recruitment to multi-national clinical studies, and the capture of real-world patient data through population-scale analyses.

Karim Ratib, MBChB, MRCP trained in interventional cardiology and transradial procedures in the West Midlands and Adelaide, Australia, before taking up an NHS consultant interventionist post at the University Hospital of North Midlands. He has a special interest in the use of radial access for complex PCI and structural heart disease.

He has a long-standing commitment to education, training, and research into the transradial technique. He participated in the development of the masterclass and centre of excellence transradial programmes at University Hospital of North Midlands and has actively supported new operators via a proctoring programme, helping to establish the technique internationally. He has published several large, highly cited studies utilising the UK national PCI database on the subject of patient outcomes related to transradial procedures, along with work related to technical improvements in the technique. He is actively engaged in access site research and was the UK principal investigator for the DISCO radial randomised study, comparing distal and conventional radial access.

He has participated in many postgraduate transradial educational and training initiatives and has been a live case operator demonstrating the radial technique.

These activities have contributed to the development, validation, and refinement of the transradial technique and the education of new operators and their teams.

Contributors

Samer Arnous
Department of Cardiology
University Hospital Limerick
Limerick, Ireland

Shrilla Banerjee
Surrey and Sussex Healthcare NHS
  Trust
East Surrey Hospital, Redhill,
  United Kingdom

Gurbir Bhatia
Department of Cardiology
Heartlands Hospital, University
  Hospitals Birmingham NHS
  Foundation Trust
Birmingham, United Kingdom

Hannah Cranch
Morriston Hospital
Swansea, United Kingdom

James Davies
Dorset County Hospital NHS
  Foundation Trust
Dorchester, Dorset, United Kingdom

Eoin Fahy
Department of Cardiology
Beaumont Hospital
Dublin, Ireland

Bethan Freestone
University Hospitals of
  Birmingham
Birmingham Heartlands Hospital
  Bordesley Green East
Birmingham, United Kingdom

Afzal Hayat
South Tees Hospitals NHS
  Foundation Trust
Tyne and Wear, United Kingdom

Cara Hendry
Manchester University NHS
  Foundation Trust
Wythenshawe Hospital, Southmoor
  United Kingdom

Jonathan Hinton
University Hospital Dorset
Bournemouth, United Kingdom

Shazia T. Hussain
Glenfield Hospital
University Hospitals of Leicester
  NHS Trust
Leicester, United Kingdom

Sophia Khattak
University of Birmingham
Birmingham, United Kingdom

Thomas Kiernan
Department of Cardiology
University Hospital Limerick
Limerick, Ireland
School of Medicine, University of
Limerick, Limerick, Ireland

Darren Klass
Interventional Radiology
Clinical Professor – University of
British Columbia
Temporary Clinical Professor of
Radiology – Cleveland Clinic
Lerner College of Medicine of
Case Western Reserve University
Cleveland Clinic London,
United Kingdom

Mamas A. Mamas
Keele University
Congleton, United Kingdom

Peter O'Kane
Dorset Heart Centre
The Royal Bournemouth Hospital
Bournemouth
Dorset, United Kingdom

Claudio Proscia
Liverpool Heart and Chest Hospital
NHS Foundation Trust
Thomas Drive, Liverpool,
United Kingdom

Sudhir Rathore
Department of Cardiology
Frimley Health NHS Foundation
Trust
Camberley, United Kingdom

Karim Ratib
University Hospital of North Midlands
Staffordshire, United Kingdom

Helen Routledge
Department of Cardiology
Worcestershire Acute Hospitals NHS
Trust
Worcester, United Kingdom

Warkaa Shamkhani
Keele Cardiovascular Research Group
Centre for Prognosis Research
Keele University
North Midlands, United Kingdom

Bing Wei Thaddeus Soh
Department of Cardiology
University Hospital Limerick
Limerick, Ireland

Rodney H. Stables
Liverpool Heart and Chest Hospital
Thomas Drive, Liverpool,
United Kingdom

David Wells
University of the North Midlands
NHS Trust
Longton Road, Stone, United Kingdom

Fraser Witherow
Dorset County Cardiac Center
Dorchester, Dorset, United Kingdom

Azfar Zaman
Freeman Hospital and Newcastle
University
Newcastle upon Tyne,
United Kingdom

Patient Selection

1

Hannah Cranch and Mamas A. Mamas

1.1 OVERVIEW OF ACCESS SITE OPTIONS

Gaining vascular access is the first technical aspect of any percutaneous procedure and is therefore crucial to performing a successful and safe procedure. The radial artery originates from the brachial artery, which bifurcates into the ulnar and radial arteries at the level of the antecubital fossa. The radial artery runs laterally in the forearm, becoming more superficial at the wrist. In the hand, it connects with the ulnar artery via extensive collaterals arising from the superficial and deep palmar arch, minimising the risk of distal limb ischaemia in the event of vascular injury/occlusion. Compared to the transfemoral artery approach (TFA), radial access is associated with a reduced risk of vascular complications, major bleeding, and mortality in high-risk cases, such as acute coronary syndromes. It has therefore been widely adopted, particularly for cardiac intervention, and is recommended as a Class 1 indication in recent guidelines [1, 2].

The radial artery has a mean diameter close to 3 mm in men and is 10%–15% smaller in women. In contrast, the femoral artery is significantly larger at around 6 mm in diameter in most patients [3]. Equipment has been miniaturised and haemostasis devices manufactured, facilitating a shift towards radial access as standard care. The brachial artery, which had previously been used for vascular access, is seldom used owing to it being procedurally more difficult and associated with a high risk of vascular and neurological complications because of its proximity to the median nerve. Haemostasis at the site of brachial artery access is also more challenging.

DOI: 10.1201/9781003153627-1

Another major advantage of transradial artery access (TRA) is that, in contrast to the femoral and ulnar arteries, the radial artery lies superficially, overlying bone in its distal portion and is therefore easier to palpate for puncturing and to compress for haemostasis. Following TFA access, patients require a one- to six-hour period of bed rest, which can be uncomfortable and often results in a longer inpatient stay. TRA removes the need for bed rest; once the arterial sheath is removed, a compression device is applied with no restrictions on patient mobility. This increases the likelihood of same-day discharge, reduces the workload for nursing staff, increases comfort, and increases patient satisfaction and cost savings.

1.2 DATA SUPPORTING THE PREFERENTIAL USE OF RADIAL ARTERY ACCESS

A large number of randomised trials have investigated the benefits of radial access compared to femoral access. The ACCESS Study in 1997 was the first randomised control trial (RCT) comparing radial, femoral and brachial artery access for percutaneous transluminal coronary angioplasty (PTCA), showing similar procedural success but reduced vascular complications with radial access [4]. Same-day discharge following TRA was demonstrated to be feasible soon after this. The RIVAL trial [5] comparing TRA and TFA in over 7,000 patients with acute coronary syndrome (ACS) showed similar procedural success for both access sites. Radial access was associated with a reduction in vascular complications and a reduction in major adverse events in higher-risk patients, such as patients presenting with ST elevation myocardial infarction (STEMI), particularly when centres performed a high volume of radial cases. A reduction in cardiac mortality associated with TRA was also observed in RIFLE-STEACS 2012 [6] in a STEMI population. A non-significant reduction in mortality with TRA was similarly observed in STEMI-RADIAL 2014 [7], which demonstrated a significant reduction in major bleeding and vascular complications. The MATRIX study is the largest multicentre RCT comparing TRA and TFA in over 8,000 ACS patients undergoing percutaneous coronary intervention (PCI). Net adverse clinical events (NACE) were significantly lower in the TRA arm of the study, driven by a reduction in major bleeding and all-cause mortality [8].

Data from the previous studies has been combined with other smaller RCTs in a meta-analysis of pooled data from over 22,000 patients. This demonstrated that radial access, compared with femoral access, was associated with a lower risk of all-cause mortality and major adverse cardiac events (MACE) across the entire spectrum of coronary artery disease and reaffirmed that TRA is associated with significantly fewer major bleeding and vascular complications [9]. This mortality benefit has also been supported by a more recent meta-analysis of seven RCTs analysed at an individual patient level, where 30-day all-cause mortality was reduced in TRA patients when compared to TFA [10]. Analysis of subsets confirms that the benefits of TRA are maximised in the highest-risk patients, such as those with increased bleeding risks, advanced age, female sex, and risk factors for TFA complications.

This extensive series of RCTs has stimulated a major and rapid change in access site practice in the UK, with most cases now performed via TRA. There remain some global variations in radial access adoption for coronary angiography and PCI, with Europe and Asia adopting TRA at higher rates than the United States. The UK national PCI database has been used to investigate outcomes in large numbers of unselected patients. The studies confirm that adoption of TRA into clinical practice has resulted in a reduction in bleeding rates and a move towards more same-day discharge related to the safety of TRA [11, 12]. There is also an increasing use of radial access for complex PCI with associated reduced length of stay, major bleeding, and vascular complications [13–15]. TRA is now used for the majority of complex cases in the UK, with TFA reserved for cases in which large-diameter guide catheters cannot be deployed via TRA.

1.3 SELECTING PATIENTS FOR TRA PROCEDURES

Given the evidence supporting TRA, it is the first choice for vascular access in most percutaneous procedures where TFA does not provide a specific advantage. Transradial artery access is associated with a higher cannulation failure rate with crossover to TFA in 5% of cases, particularly during an operator's learning curve [8]. Contributing factors to this are the radial artery having a smaller diameter, the increased incidence of anatomical variants, and the propensity for spasm in a cannulated radial. With increasing operator volume, failure rates are reduced.

Patient selection is key in ensuring TRA success. Despite TRA now being part of standard care in many PCI centres across the world, there are some patients for whom the choice would be less favourable. The factors that influence choosing the radial artery approach can be categorised as patient related, technical, and

TABLE 1.1   Factors associated with increased TRA procedural complexity

FACTORS ASSOCIATED WITH INCREASED TRA PROCEDURAL COMPLEXITY		
PATIENT-RELATED FACTORS	TECHNICAL FACTORS	ANATOMICAL FACTORS
Female Sex	Impalpable radial pulse	Known radial or subclavian anatomical anomaly
Cardiogenic shock	Previous radial failure	
Previous CABG	Need for enhanced guiding catheter support or multiple devices requiring a large-diameter guide	Abnormal aortic morphology
Fixed flexion deformity of the arm		Known radial artery occlusion
Previous severe radial spasm		
Extremes of stature		
Advanced age		

anatomical (Table 1.1). When these factors are present, a TRA procedure may be more difficult – it is a good strategy to avoid or proceed with caution in patients who have a number of these features during an operator's learning curve or if time delay due to technical complexity will be disadvantageous. More experienced operators can adopt specific strategies to enhance the chances of a successful outcome, even in these more challenging patients. Reviewing any previous angiographic images for each patient is essential as it can provide useful insights on access choice. If prior imaging demonstrates difficult guiding catheter support, a radial loop, or significant subclavian tortuosity, an alternative access site to the radial artery/contralateral radial artery may be considered.

The MATRIX score has been validated to identify those at high risk of TRA failure needing crossover using eight independent predictors: age, height, history of renal failure, previous coronary artery bypass grafts (CABG), current smoker, STEMI presentation, Killip class ≥ II, and the centre's proportion of TRA intervention. It is well recognised that the radial artery has a propensity to arterial spasm, which in some cases can be severe. When the risk of spasm is increased, pre-procedure sedation and analgesia, as well as liberal use of vasodilators, are advised. Cardiogenic shock can make radial artery cannulation more difficult, and in selected cases, patients require mechanical device support (e.g., intra-aortic balloon pump or percutaneous left ventricular support device), which would necessitate TFA to accommodate the large-diameter delivery system. Patients who have undergone previous CABG should have access via the left radial artery to ease the engagement of left internal mammary and venous grafts.

The radial artery is able to accommodate an 8 French guiding catheter within a well-sized radial artery, and so TRA is increasingly used for complex intervention. In individuals with smaller radials that cannot accommodate larger-diameter guide systems, TFA is often preferred.

1.4 CONTRAINDICATIONS/CAUTIONS

There are very few absolute contraindications to TRA (Table 1.2). Any active bleeding or infection at the radial artery cannulation site is a contraindication to vascular puncture.

Patients with an arteriovenous dialysis fistula should not have instrumentation of the ipsilateral radial artery. Radial puncture and subsequent intervention may be performed on the contralateral side with caution, as occlusion of the artery may prevent the preparation of a fistula in the future. Patients who have had breast cancer surgery are often advised to avoid vascular puncture in the upper limb on the same side as the surgery, and they may therefore be reluctant to undergo a transradial procedure. Observational series do not suggest that TRA is associated with an increased lymphoedema risk, but it is important to ensure that the patient is fully informed about relative access site risks and that their preference is respected when choosing an access site. In patients with Raynaud's disease, associated with a vasculitic systemic connective tissue disease, the collateralisation of the hand circulation may be compromised, and there are case reports of ischaemia after TRA – we recommend avoiding radial cannulation in these circumstances. Severe patient anxiety increases the risk of radial spasm. This can usually be controlled with upfront administration of intravenous sedation and anxiolytics, but if these pharmacological measures

TABLE 1.2 Contraindications and cautions to transradial artery access

CONTRAINDICATIONS	CAUTIONS
Local infection around puncture site	Pain
Pre-existing haematoma at puncture site	Uncontrolled patient anxiety
Arteriovenous dialysis fistula ipsilateral side	Previous mastectomy and axillary clearance surgery
Systemic connective tissue disorder with or without severe Raynaud's Disease	Difficulty with radial puncture in a time critical procedure (such as STEMI angioplasty)

fail, an alternative access site may be more suitable. If procedural success is time dependent and there are factors that increase TRA complexity, an alternative access site may be chosen. This is most relevant to primary angioplasty cases – it is, however, important to note that TRA in these patients has multiple advantages and significantly improves outcomes. Experienced operators can perform TRA in primary cases without prolongation of door to balloon time.

1.5 CONCLUSIONS

Transradial artery access for PCI, compared with transfemoral artery access, is associated with a lower risk of mortality, major adverse cardiovascular events, major bleeding, and vascular complications. TRA is more comfortable for the patient, allows early mobilisation, and reduces hospital stay by facilitating same-day discharge protocols. Patient selection for TRA can reduce the failure rate and need for crossover as some patients can be easily identified as at increased risk of procedural complexity. In these more complex patients, measures can be instituted to improve procedural success. For each individual patient, careful consideration is needed to identify the optimal access site, taking into consideration individual patient factors and operator experience. There are very few contraindications to TRA, and it represents the best access site choice for most patients.

REFERENCES

1. Lawton JS, Tamis-Holland JE, Bangalore S, Bates ER, Beckie TM, Bischoff JM, et al. 2021 ACC/AHA/SCAI Guideline for Coronary Artery Revascularization: Executive Summary: A Report of the American College of Cardiology/American Heart Association Joint Committee on Clinical Practice Guidelines. *J Am Coll Cardiol.* 2022;79(2):197–215.
2. Collet JP, Thiele H, Barbato E, Barthélémy O, Bauersachs J, Bhatt DL, et al. 2020 ESC Guidelines for the Management of Acute Coronary Syndromes in Patients Presenting Without Persistent ST-Segment Elevation. *Eur Heart J.* 2021;42(14):1289–1367.
3. Yoo BS, Yoon J, Ko JY, Kim JY, Lee SH, Hwang SO, et al. Anatomical Consideration of the Radial Artery for Transradial Coronary Procedures:

Arterial Diameter, Branching Anomaly and Vessel Tortuosity. *Int J Cardiol.* 2005;*101*(3):421–7.

4. Kiemeneij F, Laarman GJ, Odekerken D, Slagboom T, van der Wieken R. A Randomized Comparison of Percutaneous Transluminal Coronary Angioplasty by the Radial, Brachial and Femoral Approaches: The Access Study. *J Am Coll Cardiol.* 1997;*29*(6):1269–75.

5. Jolly SS, Yusuf S, Cairns J, Niemelä K, Xavier D, Widimsky P, et al. Radial versus Femoral Access for Coronary Angiography and Intervention in Patients With Acute Coronary Syndromes (RIVAL): A Randomised, Parallel Group, Multicentre Trial. *Lancet.* 2011;*377*(9775):1409–20.

6. Romagnoli E, Biondi-Zoccai G, Sciahbasi A, Politi L, Rigattieri S, Pendenza G, et al. Radial versus Femoral Randomized Investigation in ST-Segment Elevation Acute Coronary Syndrome: The RIFLE-STEACS (Radial Versus Femoral Randomized Investigation in ST-Elevation Acute Coronary Syndrome) Study. *J Am Coll Cardiol.* 2012;*60*(24):2481–9.

7. Bernat I, Horak D, Stasek J, Mates M, Pesek J, Ostadal P, et al. ST-Segment Elevation Myocardial Infarction Treated by Radial or Femoral Approach in a Multicenter Randomized Clinical Trial: The STEMI-RADIAL Trial. *J Am Coll Cardiol.* 2014;*63*(10):964–72.

8. Valgimigli M, Gagnor A, Calabró P, Frigoli E, Leonardi S, Zaro T, et al. Radial versus Femoral Access in Patients With Acute Coronary Syndromes Undergoing Invasive Management: A Randomised Multicentre Trial. *Lancet.* 2015;*385*(9986):2465–76.

9. Ferrante G, Rao SV, Jüni P, Da Costa BR, Reimers B, Condorelli G, et al. Radial versus Femoral Access for Coronary Interventions Across the Entire Spectrum of Patients With Coronary Artery Disease: A Meta-Analysis of Randomized Trials. *JACC Cardiovasc Interv.* 2016;*9*(14):1419–34.

10. Gargiulo G, Giacoppo D, Jolly SS, Cairns J, Le May M, Bernat I, et al. Effects on Mortality and Major Bleeding of Radial Versus Femoral Artery Access for Coronary Angiography or Percutaneous Coronary Intervention: Meta-Analysis of Individual Patient Data From 7 Multicenter Randomized Clinical Trials. *Circulation.* 2022;*146*(18):1329–43.

11. Taxiarchi P, Kontopantelis E, Martin GP, Kinnaird T, Curzen N, Banning AP, et al. Same-Day Discharge After Elective Percutaneous Coronary Intervention: Insights From the British Cardiovascular Intervention Society. *JACC Cardiovasc Interv.* 2019;*12*(15):1479–94.

12. Olier I, Carr M, Curzen N, Ludman P, Baumbach A, Kinnaird T, et al. Changes in Periprocedural Bleeding Complications Following Percutaneous Coronary Intervention in The United Kingdom Between 2006 and 2013 (From the British Cardiovascular Interventional Society). *Am J Cardiol.* 2018;*122*(6):952–60.

13. Kinnaird T, Anderson R, Gallagher S, Sharp ASP, Farooq V, Ludman P, et al. Vascular Complications Associated With Intraaortic Balloon Pump Supported Percutaneous Coronary Intervention (PCI) and Clinical Outcomes From the British Cardiovascular Intervention Society National PCI Database. *Catheter Cardiovasc Interv.* 2021;*98*(1):E53–e61.

14. Kinnaird T, Anderson R, Gallagher S, Sirker A, Ludman P, de Belder M, et al. Access Site and Outcomes for Unprotected Left Main Stem Percutaneous

Coronary Intervention: An Analysis of the British Cardiovascular Intervention Society Database. *JACC Cardiovasc Interv.* 2018;*11*(24):2480–91.

15. Kinnaird T, Cockburn J, Gallagher S, Choudhury A, Sirker A, Ludman P, et al. Temporal Changes in Radial Access Use, Associates and Outcomes in Patients Undergoing PCI Using Rotational Atherectomy Between 2007 and 2014: Results From the British Cardiovascular Intervention Society National Database. *Am Heart J.* 2018;*198*:46–54.

Patient Preparation and Cardiac Catheter Laboratory Set-up

2

Sophia Khattak and Bethan Freestone

2.1 INTRODUCTION

The first transradial coronary angiogram was performed in 1989 by Dr Lucien Campeau [1, 2]; the next 35 years have seen huge advances in devices specifically designed for radial access, as well as our understanding of technical challenges posed by issues such as variant radial anatomy. This chapter will focus on the important issues of the learning curve, pre-procedural evaluation, and strategic planning, leading to optimisation of set-up for radial procedures.

DOI: 10.1201/9781003153627-2

2.2 THE TRANSRADIAL LEARNING CURVE

For both cardiology trainees and for established femoral approach operators looking to utilise the radial artery approach for coronary angiography and percutaneous coronary intervention (PCI), there is a recognised learning curve [3]. Studies have suggested that it can take 50 to 100 procedures for an operator to become proficient at transradial coronary angiography, even if they are already an experienced femoral operator (although this may vary depending on the operator's experience and learning capabilities). Other contemporary studies suggest that the learning curve may be around 200 procedures. A structured learning programme with initial direct supervision for cases combined with specific radial operator training with mentorship, simulator training workshops, courses, peer-to-peer discussions, and feedback are methods of reducing the length of the learning curve. As with any experiential learning, it is recommended to start with simpler cases and gradually increase the complexity of the procedures as experience and skill level improve [3]. It is important to ensure that the patient is as calm as possible to minimise spasm risk. Spasm is more common during the learning curve, and use of vasodilators will help to mitigate this risk.

2.3 PATIENT PREPARATION

During the pre-procedure discussions with the patient, it is important to assess anxiety level. High levels of anxiety increase the risk of radial spasm and should be managed by proactively administering peri-procedural intravenous sedation and analgesia. Relevant comorbidities such as previous breast cancer surgery or concomitant oral anticoagulant therapy should be identified before the patient enters the catheterisation laboratory so that appropriate discussion of available access options and post-procedure care can form part of the consent process. In the presence of more advanced age or extremes of stature, consider electively using a left radial approach. The left arm is an anatomically simpler environment with less subclavian tortuosity and so can improve procedural success rates in challenging cases. An assessment of the patient's bleeding and ischaemic risk will facilitate optimal procedural and post-procedural planning. It is important to inspect the planned radial puncture site. This will identify local problems such as scars or infections, alert the operator to the presence of musculoskeletal abnormalities that may limit arm movement, and confirm the presence of a palpable pulse. If the pulse is impalpable, then a radial ultrasound can be performed to assess the potential for proceeding with a puncture or switching access site.

2.4 CARDIAC CATHETER LABORATORY PREPARATION AND SET-UP

The set-up in the cardiac catheter lab for either radial or femoral artery approach coronary angiography or PCI is similar, (as in Figure 2.1) but there are some specific aspects to consider when using the radial approach. Optimising and tailoring the laboratory set-up for radial procedures is important to ensure patient and operator comfort, for successful puncture of the radial artery and for radiation protection for the operator. A simple (as in Figure 2.1) or a specifically designed arm board (such as the Starboard shown in Figure 2.2a) can be used for radial artery procedures. The left or right arm can be used, but the right radial artery is usually preferred for most procedures, as it is more accessible and provides an optimal ergonomic position for the operator. For arterial puncture, the arm is first placed on the arm board with the wrist supported and gently extended (Figure 2.2b). The wrist is then cleaned and draped in the usual manner to achieve a sterile field. Specific drapes optimised for radial procedures which have gaps positioned to lie over the wrist area are available and simplify draping the operating field.

Under standard aseptic conditions, local anaesthesia is injected over the radial, and arterial access is gained using a modified Seldinger technique to insert a specifically designed radial artery sheath, as detailed in Section 3.5 in Chapter 3. After arterial access is gained, it is important to move the arm into a position close to the side of the patient, as this aids patient comfort and operator radiation protection. It allows the operator to stand further away from the X-ray source and facilitates deployment of correctly positioned radiation barriers, such as over- and under-table shields. It is important that the patient's arm is well supported for the case to avoid the arm drifting and that the specifically designed arm boards also have an operator "platform" attachment to help maintain an ergonomically favourable operating position, as well as offering additional radiation protection against backscatter from the patient (see Figure 2.2 for the arm board and operating positions for right and left radial access using the Starboard to support – a similar set-up can be achieved with locally customised arm board configurations).

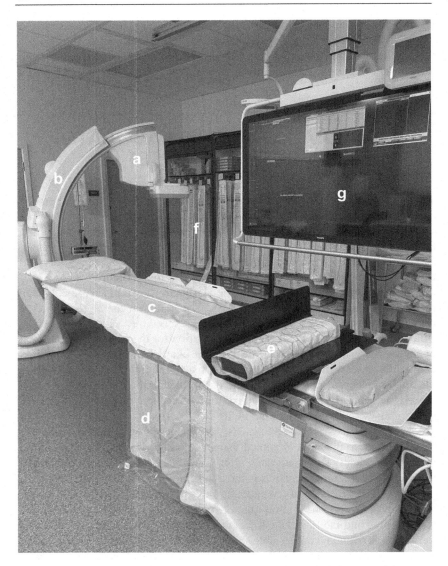

FIGURE 2.1   Catheterisation laboratory set-up. (a) Flat panel detector, (b) C arm, (c) patient table, (d) under-table protective shielding, (e) a simple arm board, (f) cabinets containing consumables, (g) display screen and monitor.

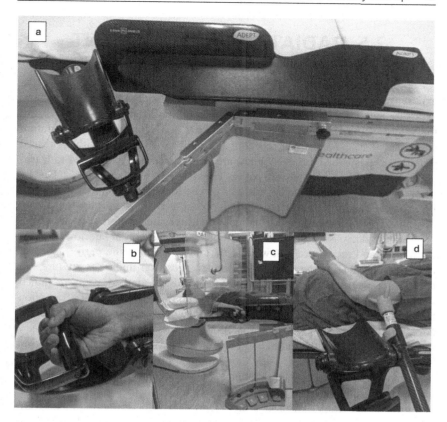

FIGURE 2.2   Arm board configuration. (a) Starboard, (b) patient position with extended wrist, (c) right radial arm position with well positioned ceiling-mounted and under-table shielding, (d) left radial arm position.

For left radial cases, the operator can choose to stay on the right hand of the table for puncturing – the patient's arm will need to be brought across the body to facilitate access to the puncture site. As an alternative, the operator can move to the left-hand side to puncture, with the patient's arm extended and abducted and supported on an arm board. Once access has been secured, using either approach, the patient's arm is positioned partially adducted over the abdomen so that the operator can access the radial introducer sheath without leaning over the patient. It is usually necessary to secure the arm with a sling or a supporting bolster to prevent it from dropping back to the patient's left-hand side during the procedure.

2.5 RADIATION MANAGEMENT

As coronary angiography and PCI involve the use of X-ray imaging, this exposes patients and health-care professionals to ionising radiation. Minimising exposure and good radiation protection are essential in the cath lab to ensure the safety of patients and health-care workers. Early observational literature suggested that radial access procedures could be associated with increased radiation exposure. Much of the measured difference may be related to learning curve issues and mismatched patient characteristics in these studies. During an operator's learning curve, procedures can be longer and require more imaging, so particular attention needs to be applied to radiation protection during this phase. More recent studies indicate that measured differences in current practice are decreasing or have been abolished. This may relate to improved equipment and procedural knowledge that has simplified the performance of radial cases, reducing the need for prolonged, radiation-intense procedures. In addition, as the radial technique has been studied and applied, we have gained more knowledge relating to radial-specific methods of optimising radiation protection, and it is important to ensure that we apply these techniques. Close attention to optimised radiation protection ensures that experienced coronary interventionists using the radial approach do not have any increase in radiation exposure when compared to using the femoral approach [4].

Appropriate protective equipment, such as lead aprons and thyroid collars, are worn by all personnel in the room. In addition to standard protective clothing, further radiation protection, such as lead glasses and shinpads, are effective in reducing exposure and should be worn for all cases (Figure 2.3). The data supporting currently available caps is conflicting, and they are not proven to decrease operator brain exposure. For female operators, additional shielding devices are available that can be applied to the upper arm to provide enhanced protection to breast tissue contained within the axilla.

Although total protection systems are available (such as the Rampart system), these are not currently available in most laboratories. Conventional barrier shielding devices, such as an under-table shield and ceiling-mounted shield, are very effective at reducing operator radiation exposure when properly utilised. The over-table shield should be positioned close to the patient and in contact with their body to minimise backscatter exposure. Other radiation reduction measures, such as drapes on the patient (e.g., Radpad), further limit backscatter exposure. An upward projecting radiation shield attached to the armboard in commercially available systems, like the Starboard, will close the gap between over-table and under-table shields and directly applied drapes, providing optimal operator shielding for radial procedures.

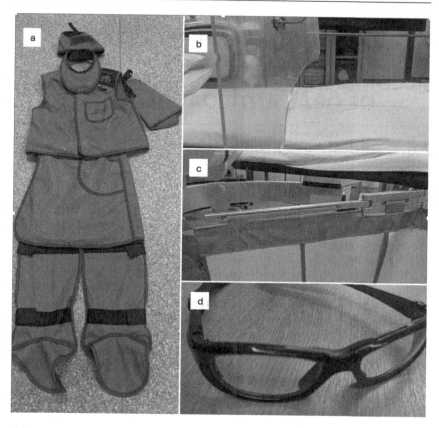

FIGURE 2.3 Radiation protection. (a) Personal protective clothing with additional hat, thyroid shield, arm shield and shinpads, (b) ceiling-mounted shield, (c) under-table shielding, (d) lead glasses.

It is important to employ good standard radiation practice as per ionising radiation medical exposure regulations (IRMER), limit the duration and frequency of fluoroscopy/acquisitions, and ensure the appropriate use of collimation and filters. Maximising the distance between the X-ray source and the operator reduces exposure by the inverse square law, so extension tubing on the manifold can be used to allow the operator to move further away from the X-ray source. Real-time radiation monitoring (e.g., DoseAware, Philips) in the cath lab allows radiation exposure to be measured and can be used to identify areas where exposure levels can be reduced.

2.6 PRE- AND PERI-PROCEDURE PHARMACOLOGY (INCLUDING RECOMMENDATIONS ON MANAGEMENT OF ORAL ANTICOAGULATION)

2.6.1 Radial "Cocktail"

After radial artery sheath insertion, it has been standard practice to give a mixture of medications through the radial sheath. This is known as a radial "cocktail." Firstly, to reduce spasm in the radial artery, vasodilators such as nitrates or verapamil can be given (particularly when using shorter sheaths where radial artery spasm can hamper progress). Secondly, anticoagulation with heparin, at a dose of 5,000 units, is recommended, as this has been shown to reduce the risk of radial artery occlusion post-procedurally [5]. More details on these drug strategies are provided in Section 3.4. Experienced operators have fewer problems with radial spasm. They often elect to reserve vasodilators until clinically apparent spasm or anatomical challenges are encountered. If a radial cocktail containing heparin is administered through the sheath-side arm, then the low pH of the heparin is likely to cause discomfort. It is important to minimise this by drawing some blood back into the drug administration syringe, as mixing will raise the pH of the solution – the patient should also be warned of possible brief discomfort.

2.6.2 Antiplatelet Therapy

Whether patients are undergoing diagnostic coronary angiography and proceeding to PCI via a radial artery or a femoral artery route, most patients will have been pre-treated with antiplatelet agents. Aspirin is currently given as standard treatment in almost all patients undergoing PCI (unless the patient has true aspirin allergy or in some high-risk bleeding patients on anticoagulants). Dual antiplatelet therapy, with a P2Y12 blocker as the second antiplatelet agent, is administered for PCI [6], and this combination therapy with more potent antiplatelet agents can further increase bleeding risks, enhancing the potential benefits of radial access [7]. The use of glycoprotein IIb/IIIa inhibitors (GPI) for enhanced platelet inhibition is usually reserved for bailout in slow flow or no flow or where the thrombus load is high, but not usually for stable angina patients undergoing PCI because they have shown no mortality benefit (but non-fatal MIs are shown to be reduced) [8]. The use of more effective antiplatelet therapy, plus the need for peri-procedural anticoagulation for PCI with unfractionated heparin, increases the risk of access site bleeding in PCI. The need for additional antithrombotic treatments, such as GPIs, incrementally increases bleeding risk, particularly in acute coronary syndrome patients. The risk of access site bleeding is significant in ACS patients and is reduced by using the radial approach as compared to the femoral approach, resulting in improved clinical outcomes [9].

2.6.3 Anticoagulation

Patients undergoing cardiac catheterisation are frequently treated with oral anticoagulants for stroke prevention in atrial fibrillation (AF), for treatment of previous venous thromboembolism, or as an essential treatment for mechanical heart valves. In ST elevation myocardial infarction (STEMI), coronary intervention cannot be delayed; therefore, radial approach primary PCI carries a reduced bleeding risk when compared to the femoral artery approach, particularly in anticoagulated patients. In patients presenting with NSTEMI, anyone on a direct oral anticoagulant (DOAC) should have this stopped at least 24 hours pre-procedure (and will be without anticoagulation for a time period dependent on the half-life of the drug; see Table 2.1). This may need to be switched to low molecular weight heparin in patients at high risk of thromboembolism if the time to coronary angiography and PCI is delayed. For patients on warfarin, coronary angiography and/or PCI is considered safe via the radial approach even at therapeutic INR [10]. In these patients, close attention to haemostasis with a prolonged compression time will be needed. In comparison, the INR should be less than 1.6 if using a femoral artery approach.

TABLE 2.1   Pharmacology of frequently used direct oral anticoagulants

DRUG	DABIGATRAN	APIXABAN	RIVAROXABAN	EDOXABAN
Mechanism of action	Direct thrombin inhibitor	Factor Xa inhibitor	Factor Xa inhibitor	Factor Xa inhibitor
Half-life	12–14 h	8–15 h	5–13 h	10–14 h
Dose in AF	150 mg or 110 mg bd	5 mg bd or 2.5 mg bd	20 mg or 15 mg od	60 mg od
Important drug interactions	Verapamil – reduce dose			Verapamil – reduce dose

After any PCI, for patients on anticoagulation, an assessment of bleeding risk versus ischaemic and stroke risk should be considered. The European Society of Cardiology (ESC) guidelines recommend triple therapy with aspirin, clopidogrel, and a DOAC for one week as a default strategy, but this can be prolonged for up to one month in patients with a high ischaemic risk (with a Class IIa C recommendation), after which the aspirin is usually stopped [11].

TABLE 2.2   Pre- and peri-procedural medications

DRUG	MECHANISM OF ACTION	DOSE
Aspirin	COX 2 inhibitor – Antiplatelet	300 mg loading dose followed by 75 mg od
Clopidogrel	P2Y$_{12}$ inhibitor – Antiplatelet	300–600 mg loading dose followed by 75 mg od
Prasugrel	P2Y$_{12}$ inhibitor – Antiplatelet	60 mg loading dose followed by 10 mg od (contraindicated if history of previous stroke)
Ticagrelor	P2Y$_{12}$ inhibitor – Antiplatelet	180 mg loading dose followed by 90 mg bd (contraindicated if previous cerebral haemorrhage)
Fondaparinux	Factor Xa inhibitor – Anticoagulant	2.5 mg subcutaneously for up to 8 days or until discharge. Avoid if Cr clearance <30
Enoxaparin	Low Molecular Weight Heparin – Anticoagulant	1 mg/kg subcutaneously bd for up to 8 days (reduce dose in renal impairment)
Heparin	Unfractionated heparin Anticoagulant	70–100 units/kg for PCI (Target ACT of 200–300s)
Bivalirudin	Direct thrombin inhibitor Anticoagulant	
Tirofiban	Glycoprotein inhibitor– Antiplatelet	25 mcg/kg over 3 minutes (IV high dose bolus) and then 0.15 mcg/kg/min for up to 18 hours. In patients with CrCl ≤60 mL/min give 25 mcg/kg over 3 minutes and then 0.075 mcg/kg/min
Abciximab	Glycoprotein inhibitor- Antiplatelet	0.25 mg/kg over 10–60 minutes (IV high dose bolus) and then 0.125 mcg/kg/min for 12 hours.
Eptifibatide	Glycoprotein inhibitor- Antiplatelet	180 mcg/kg over 1–2 minutes (IV high dose bolus) followed by 2 mcg/kg/min infusion. In patients with CrCl ≤60 mL/min give a reduced 1 mcg/kg/min infusion after the loading dose.

In patients at high bleeding risk, dual therapy with clopidogrel and DOAC for 6 months (instead of 12 months) is recommended. The use of the more potent P2Y12 inhibitors is not recommended with a DOAC due to increased risk of bleeding when used in patients needing double or triple antithrombotic therapy [12]. Clopidogrel has the most evidence across trials with consistently lower bleeding risk when used as antiplatelet therapy alongside an anticoagulant [13].

Table 2.2 summarises the current pre- and peri-procedural antiplatelet and antithrombotic therapies that may be used for PCI.

2.7 CONCLUSIONS

During an operator's learning curve, procedural duration and imaging requirement will be increased. In this phase, new radial operators are advised to select patients who should be less challenging for their initial cases. Careful pre-procedural assessment should help to identify important issues before the patient enters the catheterisation laboratory; this will facilitate proactive steps to minimise anxiety, guide the preferential use of left radial access, and prompt ultrasound assessment. An optimised set-up of shielding options and appropriate IRMER practices will reduce operator radiation exposure. A careful assessment of each individual patient's bleeding and ischaemic risk will serve to optimise peri- and post-procedure pharmacological management.

REFERENCES

1. Campeau L. Percutaneous Radial Artery Approach for Coronary Angiography. *Cathet Cardiovasc Diagn.* 1989;*16*(1):3–7.
2. Bertrand OF, Rao SV, Pancholy S, Jolly SS, Rodés-Cabau J, Larose É, et al. Transradial Approach for Coronary Angiography and Interventions. *JACC Cardiovasc Interv.* 2010;*3*(10):P5123.
3. Hess CN, Peterson ED, Neely ML, Dai D, Hillegass WB, Krucoff MW, et al. The Learning Curve for Transradial Percutaneous Coronary Intervention Among Operators in the United States. *Circulation.* 2014;*129*(22).
4. Becher T, Behnes M, Ünsal M, Baumann S, El-Battrawy I, Fastner C, Kuschyk C, Papavassiliu T, Hoffmann U, Mashayekhi K, Borggrefe M, Akin I. Radiation Exposure and Contrast Agent Use Related to Radial versus Femoral Arterial Access During Percutaneous Coronary Intervention (PCI)—Results of the FERARI Study. *Cardiovasc Revasc Med* 2016;*17*(8):505–509.

5. Rashid M, Kwok CS, Pancholy S, Chugh S, Kedev SA, Bernat I, Ratib K, Large A, Fraser D, Nolan J, Mamas MA. Radial Artery Occlusion After Transradial Interventions: A Systematic Review and Meta-Analysis. *J Am Heart Assoc.* 2016;*5*(1):e002686.

6. Widimský P, Motovská Z, Šimek S, Kala P, Pudil R, Holm F, et al. Clopidogrel Pre-treatment in Stable Angina: For all Patients >6 h Before Elective Coronary Angiography or Only for Angiographically Selected Patients a Few Minutes Before PCI? A Randomized Multicentre Trial PRAGUE-8. *Eur Heart J.* 2008;*29*(12): 1475–1477.

7. Neumann FJ, Sousa-Uva M, Ahlsson A, Alfonso F, Banning AP, Benedetto U, et al. 2018 ESC/EACTS Guidelines on Myocardial Revascularization, *Eur Heart J.* 2019;*40*:87–165.

8. Winchester DE, Wen X, Brearley WD, Park KE, Anderson RD, Bavry AA. Efficacy and Safety of Glycoprotein IIb/IIIa Inhibitors During Elective Coronary Revascularization: A Meta-Analysis of Randomized Trials Performed in the Era of Stents and Thienopyridines. *J Am Coll Cardiol.* 2011;*57*(10):1190–1199.

9. Jolly SS, Yusuf S, Cairns J, et al. Radial versus Femoral Access for Coronary Angiography and Intervention in Patients With Acute Coronary Syndromes (RIVAL): A Randomised, Parallel Group, Multicentre Trial. *Lancet.* 2011;*377*:1409–1420.

10. Hildick-Smith DJ, Walsh JT, Lowe MD, Petch MC. Coronary Angiography in the Fully Anticoagulated Patient: The Transradial Route Is Successful and Safe. *Catheter Cardiovasc Interv.* 2003;*58*(1):8–10.

11. Byrne RA, Rossello X, Coughlan JJ, Barbato E, Berry C, et al. 2023 ESC Guidelines for the management of Acute Coronary Syndromes. *Eur Heart J.* 2023;*44*:3720–3826

12. Sarafoff N, Martischnig A, Wealer J, Mayer K, Mehilli J, Sibbing D, et al. Triple Therapy With Aspirin, Prasugrel, and Vitamin K Antagonists in Patients With Drug-Eluting Stent Implantation and an Indication for Oral Anticoagulation. *J Am Coll Cardiol.* 2013;*61*(20):2060–2066.

13. Dewilde WJM, Oirbans T, Verheugt FWA, Kelder JC, de Smet BJGL, Herrman JP, et al. Use of Clopidogrel With or Without Aspirin in Patients Taking Oral Anticoagulant Therapy and Undergoing Percutaneous Coronary Intervention: An Open-Label, Randomised, Controlled Trial. *Lancet.* 2013;*381*(9872);1107–1115.

Radial Cannulation

3

Warkaa Shamkhani and Peter O'Kane

3.1 INTRODUCTION

Transradial arterial access (TRA) for percutaneous coronary intervention (PCI) is associated with lower bleeding and vascular complications compared to transfemoral arterial access (TFA) and is, not surprisingly, the preferred PCI access strategy in contemporary practice. The safety and efficacy of TRA are dependent on successful cannulation of the radial artery. Whilst straightforward in the vast majority of cases, this aspect of the procedure does require some thought and the purpose of this chapter is to outline the steps needed for successful cannulation.

3.2 PATIENT SELECTION

As outlined in Chapter 1, there are a small number of contraindications that should prompt the operator to consider an alternative access site. Other than this numerically small group of patients, a TRA approach is recommended for most patients undergoing diagnostic or therapeutic cardiac catheterisation.

DOI: 10.1201/9781003153627-3

3.3 PRE-PROCEDURE ASSESSMENT

Assessment of the radial artery (RA) pulse, ideally prior to the catheter lab, is important to decide whether the right or left approach is favoured. As outlined in Section 2.4, Right TRA (RRA) is often preferred for operator comfort and due to catheter lab radiation protection set-up. Left TRA (LRA) is preferable in the presence of surgical coronary bypass grafts or in older patients where there may be less anatomical variation in the forearm and subclavian vessels on the left side, reducing anticipated procedural complexity.

Simple palpation of the RA is usually sufficient to gauge the likelihood of successful puncture but of historical interest is the use of the Allen Test (AT) or Modified Allen Test (MAT) to confirm the patency of a dual arterial circulation to the hand.

First described by Edgar Van Nuys Allen in 1929, [1] this simple test confirms the presence of an intact palmar arch. In the original description, both hands were examined simultaneously, with the patient instructed to make a tight fist for 1 minute to squeeze blood out of the hand. Then during compression of either the radial or ulnar artery, the flow to the hand would be evaluated through the uncompressed artery. When the patient rapidly extended their fingers, the pallor was soon replaced by rubor with an intact circulation described as a positive AT. Persistence of pallor would suggest abnormal circulation and hence a negative AT.

A modification was suggested by Irvine Wright in 1952, with one hand examined at a time. [2] In addition, the patient elevated the hand with the fist clenched to induce pallor. The examiner compressed both radial and ulnar arteries simultaneously with their thumbs, and then the patient lowered and opened the hand slowly. As the examiner released pressure over one of the arteries, the return of rubor was assessed, as with the original AT. Under optimal conditions, it was concluded that prolonged blanching of >6 seconds is unusual in normal subjects, raising suspicion of partial or total occlusion of the artery under evaluation. [2] Pallor persistence in patches led examiners to believe there was an insufficiency of smaller vessels.

A comparison of MAT combined with plethysmography (PL) and pulse oximetry (OX) in 1,010 patients referred for coronary procedures was performed by Barbeau et al. [3] They divided the PL readings during radial compression into four types: (A) no damping, (B) slight damping of pulse trace, (C) loss followed by recovery, or (D) no recovery of pulse race within 2 minutes. OX results were either positive or negative. MAT results ≤9 seconds on either hand were observed in 93.7% patents, so 6.3% were therefore excluded from TRA. PL and OX types A, B, or C, on either hand, were observed in

98.5% of patients. Therefore, the use of PL and OX improved the sensitivity of MAT with only 1.5% cases excluded from TRA.

The adoption of PL and OX to evaluate patients prior to TRA was subsequently used in many centres to screen out the small volume of patients not suitable for TRA based on this protocol. A reverse Barbeau test (i.e., after ulnar artery compression) was also adopted after the procedure to screen for the patency of the previously instrumented RA. In cases of pattern D readings, RA occlusion could be confirmed on duplex echocardiographic examination.

The routine evaluation of collateral palmar circulation was questioned again nearly a decade later by Valgimigli et al. [4] The RADAR (Should Intervention Through Radial Approach be Denied to Patients with Negative Allen's Test Results) study was a single-centre prospective trial designed to evaluate safety and feasibility of TRA in patients with abnormal AT compared to normal AT. Two hundred three patients were selected after 942 were referred for TRA coronary procedures. They underwent several tests, including MAT, PL, and OX, thumb capillary lactate assessment at several time points, ulnar frame count, and handgrip strength tests. After initial AT, the patients were assigned into three cohorts with 83 normal (≤5 seconds), 60 intermediate (6–10 seconds), and 60 abnormal (≥10 seconds) AT results, respectively. PL pattern D (no recovery of pulse trace within 2 minutes) was recorded in 40% of abnormal AT cohorts prior to TRA. Despite this, capillary thumb lactate or hand grip strength did not differ between the groups pre- or post-TRA.

The ulnar frame count was significantly affected by the pre-procedural AT result. Patients with normal compared with those with abnormal pre-procedural AT results displayed significantly lower ulnar frame counts, suggestive of greater ulnar blood flow, post arterial sheath insertion. Although the difference in ulnar frame counts persisted after TRA across the three AT groups, there was a distinct and significant post-procedural improvement (i.e., a count reduction) only in patients with baseline abnormal AT results.

It was interesting that the patency of the ulnopalmar arches of the hand varied over time in patients who underwent TRA, with those showing less prominent ulnar and ulnopalmar collateralisation (i.e., patients with intermediate or abnormal AT results) displaying improvements after TRA. For instance, 40% PL pattern D in the AT-negative group dropped to 10% at 24 hours.

This comprehensive study therefore concluded that the patency of the ulnopalmar arches of the hand is highly dynamic, and vascular reserve inherent in the hand circulation can be recruited during and after TRA, especially in patients with poor collateral circulation at baseline. Consequently, such physiological adaptation prevents detectable objective and subjective signs of hand ischaemia during and after TRA. As a result, normal AT results are now no longer necessary before the selection of patients who can undergo TRA procedures.

3.4 PHARMACOLOGY

Standard pharmacology management of patients with either stable or acute coronary syndromes applies when TRA is adopted. However, particular consideration of analgesia and sedation is important to reduce the occurrence of RA spasm and improve successful cannulation and subsequent case completion. In addition, procedural anticoagulation is critical to prevent radial artery occlusion (RAO).

3.4.1 Anti-Spasmodics

Reducing discomfort and patient anxiety helps prevent stimulation of central neural pathways and arterial vasoconstriction. Before instrumentation of the RA, intravenous administration of benzodiazepines (Midazolam or Diazepam), either monotherapy or combined with opiates (Fentanyl or diamorphine), is highly effective in reducing patient discomfort. This clinical pathway was tested in a 2013 study of patients randomised to either sedation at the beginning of the procedure, during the preparation of the access site (Fentanyl 0.5 mg/kg and midazolam 1 mg slow intravenous push over 2 minutes), or control where no sedation was allowed [5]. In the treatment group, one additional dose was allowed 45–60 min after the first one (additional dosing according to the sedation status of the patient was not allowed because achieving "conscious sedation" status was not a requisite). The respiration rate and oxygen saturations of the patient were constantly monitored by a dedicated interventional trained nurse. These measures are particularly helpful during an operator's learning curve. Experienced operators may elect to reserve intravenous sedation and analgesia for those patients with high anxiety levels.

Radial spasm occurred in 2.6% of the treatment group versus 8.3% of control subjects ($p < 0.001$; odds ratio [OR]: 0.29). Number needed to treat (NTN) to avoid one case of spasm was 18 (95% confidence interval [CI]: 12.9 to 26.6), and the access site crossover rate was 34% lower in the treatment group: 9.9% versus 15.0% (OR: 0.62; 95% CI: 0.48 to 0.82). Patient discomfort using a visual analogue scale score was significantly lower (18.8 ± 12.5) in the treatment group compared to control subjects (27.4 ± 17.4). There were no significant differences observed in the 30-day rate of death or repeat hospital stay for any cause: 4.6% versus 4.5% (OR: 1.02; 95% CI: 0.67 to 1.56).

For the TRA site, the pre-puncture administration of topical lidocaine will further reduce pain associated with RA cannulation and sheath insertion. A small study of 76 patients randomised TRA patients to either an eutectic mixture of local anaesthesia (EMLA) cream or control prior to subsequent lidocaine infiltration, cannulation, and sheath insertion [6]. The results showed that radial pain was significantly lower in the EMLA group with blunting of the sympathetic response based on systolic blood pressure.

Further protection against radial spasm can be achieved with a "radial cocktail" using intra-arterial (IA) vasodilators after sheath insertion. Spasmolytic agents can be used with each catheter exchange or before sheath removal, although the optimal agent or combination of agents is yet to be defined. Options administered intra-arterially include Nitroglycerin (NTG) 100–200 mcg or Verapamil 2.5–5 mg. A meta-analysis concluded that Verapamil, with or without NTG, was the most effective and frequently used spasmodic agent [7].

Occasionally useful but less commonly utilised are local NTG (0.5 ml of 1% can be mixed with lidocaine) infiltration or sublingual nitrate. Vasodilators may need to be avoided or used in smaller doses in certain patients, such as those with hypotension, inferior myocardial infarction with suspected right ventricular involvement, severely impaired left ventricular ejection fraction, or severe aortic stenosis.

3.4.2 Anticoagulation

For diagnostic coronary angiography, unfractionated heparin at a dosage of 50 U/kg up to 5,000 Units is commonly used. Ideally, this is not given via the RA sheath because of potential pain and radial spasm that can develop. During PCI, higher doses of heparin (usually 70–100 U/kg) will be necessary, with the total dose dependent on the duration of the procedure. Equivalent doses of enoxaparin or bivalirudin can be used as alternatives. Patients on oral anticoagulation (OA) with either warfarin or direct oral anticoagulant (DOAC) would usually have this discontinued for the procedure, and heparin administration is identical compared to those not on OA. In the minority of cases of TRA procedures with the patients maintained on OA, heparin administration is still recommended. Definitive data on optimal procedural anticoagulation in these patients is not available – most operators empirically administer a reduced heparin dose in these circumstances.

3.5 CANNULATION TECHNIQUES

Radial cannulation can either be performed with the classical Seldinger technique or the Modified Seldinger technique whereby the guidewire is placed over a fine catheter rather than through the needle used to make the puncture.

These techniques were compared in a randomised study of 412 patients with the conclusion that the Seldinger technique was faster and more predictable than the modified version with no increase in bleeding or RAO. [8] The following approach to RA cannulation is therefore recommended:

a. Ensure the patient is properly positioned on the catheter lab table and is comfortable.
b. Extend their arm palm up with a small degree of rotation so the RA is easily palpable.
c. Clean the insertion site using antiseptic solution.
d. Consider the use of IV sedation and local anaesthesia as described.
e. Insert a 21 to 22-gauge needle (bevel upward) into the radial artery at a shallow angle until the anterior RA wall is punctured and pulsatile blood flow through the needle is achieved.
f. Alternatively, a double-wall puncture can be undertaken where the posterior RA wall is targeted with loss of pulsatile flow then observed as the needle is slightly withdrawn.
g. Once arterial placement is confirmed, advance a flexible guidewire through the needle into the arterial lumen and withdraw the needle.
h. Over the guidewire, introduce the arterial sheath with its dilator to facilitate smooth entry into the RA and then remove the dilator.
i. With the haemostatic valve on the sheath, subsequent guidewires and catheters can be advanced to the coronary circulation without any difficulty (see Chapter 4).

3.6 OPTIMISING TRA

There are two ways to optimise TRA puncture to ensure success.

3.6.1 Optimal Landmark-Based Assessment (Figure 3.1)

This technique involves locating the knowledge of the anatomy, but success varies with operator experience. An ideal position of entry is approximately 2 cm proximal to the radial styloid. If the first puncture is unsuccessful, it is often more helpful to attempt a second puncture from a more proximal position, where there is often a stronger pulsation. The operator needs to be wary

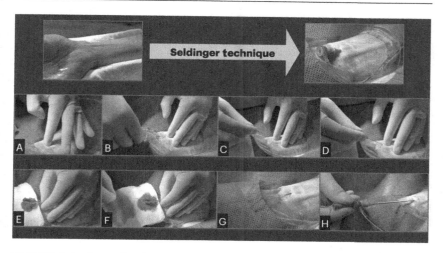

FIGURE 3.1 Steps for RA cannulation using anatomical landmarks. Panel A Palpation of radial pulse 2 cm from radial styloid; Panel B Infiltration of lidocaine (minimal initially to avoid masking landmarks); Panels C & D Radial 21G needle angled at 30–45 degrees; Panel E Successful anterior wall puncture with arterial flashback; Panels F & G Radial wire advanced through needle; Panel H Radial Glidesheath advanced over radial wire.

of a "mobile" artery whereby the needle slides across the surface rather than penetrating the wall. In these circumstances a double-wall puncture technique might be recommended to transfix the vessel initially and gain luminal access by gentle retraction of the needle.

3.6.2 Ultrasound-Guided Assessment (Figure 3.2)

Given that the RA is a relatively small vessel (usually between 2.4 mm and 2.6 mm in diameter), the ability to discriminate with fingertip palpation alone can be limited. In situations where RA is even smaller, collapsible, calcified, excessively mobile, surrounded by veins, or associated with anatomic anomalies, the landmark-analysis guided puncture technique is more likely to fail completely or significantly delay the procedure. When the PCI is time critical, such as in the setting of primary PCI for acute myocardial infarction (AMI), such delays can have a direct impact on patient outcome.

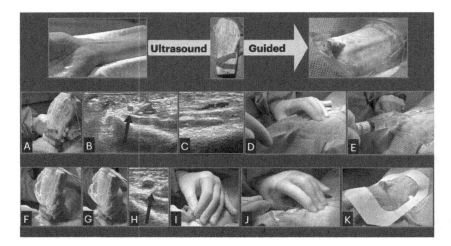

FIGURE 3.2 Steps for RA cannulation using ultrasound guidance. Panel A. Handsfree ultrasound probe positioned over RA; Panel B. Axial view of RA; Panel C. Longitudinal view RA with colour flow; Panel D. Lidocaine infiltration; Panel E. Nitrate infiltration to vasodilate (optional); Panels F-H. Radial 21G needle angled at 30–45 degrees and centrally aligned with ultrasound probe to advance to RA (arrow); Panel I. Successful anterior wall puncture with arterial flashback; Panel J. Radial wire advanced through needle; Panel K. Radial Glidesheath secured with transparent dressing.

Real-time ultrasound (US) guidance may offer a solution in these circumstances. US has been shown to be both safe and effective in cannulation of central veins [9] and for the femoral artery. [10] Indeed, such an approach is often mandated in many contemporary guidelines.

US-guided puncture can be performed using the following steps:

a. Keep the ultrasound probe in close proximity to or directly over the needle.
b. Utilise the centre mark of the ultrasound probe to align the RA with the centreline in the cross-sectional (axial plane) view.
c. Enhance needle tip identification and visualise needle movement by executing brief jabs on the skin.
d. Apply skin compression to obstruct veins and facilitate puncture precision.

The RAUST Trial (Radial Arterial Access With Ultrasound) was a prospective, multicentre randomised controlled trial that compared US-guided with palpation-guided TRA in 698 patients undergoing a radial procedure in six interventional centres. [11] The study used US machines with a high-frequency linear array transducer capable of imaging and displaying at a depth of 2 mm with a screen of at least 12.1 diagonal inches. The operators who randomised patients had minimal experience with 100 TRA cardiac procedures, with at least 15 of these US guided.

Patients received conscious sedation and had either 5F or 6F sheaths inserted with local lidocaine. A minimum of 2,000 IU unfractionated heparin or bivalirudin equivalent was used with a minimum of either 2.5 mg Verapamil or 100 mg NG to prevent spasm. Single- or double-wall puncture was left to operator discretion, and the cohort randomised to US guided had this performed as described earlier.

The results demonstrated that the number of attempts for RA puncture was significantly reduced in the US-guided group (mean: 1.65 ± 1.2 vs. 3.05 ± 3.4, $p < 0.0001$; median: 1 (interquartile range [IQR]: 1 to 2) vs. 2 (1 to 3), $p < 0.0001$). First-pass success rate improved (64.8% vs. 43.9%, $p < 0.0001$) with US guidance. The time to access was also reduced (88 ± 78 seconds vs. 108 ± 112 seconds, $p = 0.006$; median: 64 [IQR: 45 to 94] seconds vs. 74 [IQR: 49 to 120] seconds, $p = 0.01$). Ten patients in the control group required crossover to US guidance after 5 min of failed palpation attempts, with 8 of 10 (80%) having successful sheath insertion with US. The number of difficult access procedures was decreased with US guidance (2.4% vs. 18.6% for ≥ 5 attempts, $p < 0.001$; 3.7% vs. 6.8% for ≥ 5 min, $p = 0.07$). There was no significant difference observed in the rate of operator-reported spasm, patient pain scores following the procedure, or bleeding complications.

US-guided TRA, at least from this trial, would appear to provide higher TRA success in cannulation with fewer overall attempts, a higher first-pass rate, and a 20-second time reduction [11]. Given this data, it is recommended that operators become familiar with US guidance and incorporate this into their routine practice.

3.7 ACCESS WIRE AND SHEATH SELECTION

Careful selection of sheaths and access wires is important to ensure procedural safety and efficacy after TRA cannulation. Sheaths come in various types and sizes, and selection requires a balance between procedural efficiency and the risk of access site complications. Typical radial sheaths feature a tapered-tip dilator that allows for smooth passage within the vessel. Hydrophilic-coated sheaths were thought to reduce arterial spasm and increase patient comfort, but their usage has declined in recent years. Whilst efficacious, occasional access site dermal sterile granulomas caused by coating removal during sheath insertion were troublesome [12].

The use of 5 Fr sheaths can lead to fewer complications than using 6 Fr sheaths. A smaller sheath-to-artery ratio is favoured to minimise the risk of RAO. Studies indicate an increased risk of occlusion when the sheath diameter exceeds 1.0 times the RA diameter (4.0% vs. 13%, $p = 0.0113$) [13].

Generally, a 6 Fr sheath is well-tolerated, but for smaller patients and women who are more prone to RAO, starting with a 5 Fr sheath is advised, allowing for an upgrade to 6 Fr if PCI becomes necessary. However, contemporary radial sheaths (5 Fr or 6 Fr) can accommodate diagnostic or guide catheters with outer diameters of 6 Fr or 7 Fr, respectively, so this upgrade is no longer necessary. For example, Glidesheath Slender (Terumo, Japan) maintains a wider inner diameter with the same outer diameter, which enhances procedural flexibility for TRA interventions. Most PCI can be performed through 6F guiding systems, but certain procedures – e.g., large burr rotational atherectomy, retrograde conduit CTO techniques, and some two-stent left main bifurcation techniques – are more easily performed with 7F guides.

Radial sheaths also come in flexible lengths of 10–13 cm and 23–25 cm. Rathore et al. performed a prospective, randomised, 2 × 2 factorial designed, study of short (13 cm) sheath versus long (23 cm) sheath and hydrophilic-coated versus uncoated sheaths in 790 patients. [14] Procedural success was achieved in 96% of the cases, and RA spasm accounted for 17 of 33 failed cases. Interestingly, there was significantly less RA spasm (19.0% vs. 39.9%, odds ratio [OR]: 2.87; 95% confidence interval [CI]: 2.07 to 3.97, $p < 0.001$) and patient-reported discomfort (15.1% vs. 28.5%, OR: 2.27; 95% CI: 1.59 to 3.23, $p < 0.001$) in patients receiving a hydrophilic-coated sheath. However, there was no difference observed between short and long sheaths. RAO, which was relatively high in this study, was observed in 9.5% of patients but was not accounted for by sheath selection [14].

The outcomes of different sheath sizes in TRA have been studied in a number of clinical trials. An alternative approach to a conventional sheath involves the use of a sheathless guide, discussed in greater detail in Section 5.5.5. The 7.5-F sheathless guide has a smaller outer diameter compared to a 6-F regular sheath. Additionally, its inner diameter of 0.081 inches allows for the passage of a wider range of interventional equipment, such as a large burr rotablator. However, these guides are not widely adopted in practice due to their comparative inflexibility (stiffness) and limited shape range. The Railway Sheathless Access System is an innovative device that converts preferred guiding catheters into a sheathless access system. This provides a smaller access profile, enables tracking through radial anatomy with or without a sheath, and reduces the risk of spasm and RAO. The device is compatible with hundreds of guiding catheters and comes in versatile 5F, 6F, and 7F sizes. Catheter-assisted tracking (see Chapter 7) can also be used to facilitate the deployment of conventional guides via a sheathless approach.

Access wires, crucial for guiding sheath and then subsequent catheters, have their own set of selection criteria to consider and are discussed further in Chapter 4. After needle cannulation, it may be helpful to use a standard 0.014″ PCI wire if the dedicated sheath wire (usually 0.018″) does not track. Similarly, when encountering more hostile distal radial anatomy such as tortuosity or spasm, wiring all the way to the aorta with the 0.014″ can facilitate subsequent catheter exchange for a standard 0.035″ guidewire. An early bifurcation of the radial can similarly prevent easy access of the guidewire and catheter, and clear evidence of a recurrent RA path may prompt a switch to an alternative access site. Any resistance to 6F or 5F catheter passage can be assisted with an inner 5F or 4F catheter (catheter-assisted tracking – CAT) or use of balloon-assisted tracking (BAT) outlined in Chapter 4.

3.8 RECOGNISING AND DEALING WITH IMMEDIATE COMPLICATIONS

The successful performance of TRA procedures relies on an in-depth understanding of potential complications and the implementation of effective mitigation strategies. Common complications are as follows.

3.8.1 Radial Artery Spasm

RA spasm complicates procedures, hindering catheter advancement and potentially causing pain, dissection, and occasionally perforation. Mitigation of radial spasm requires the following considerations:

- Obtain an arm angiogram to identify variant anatomy that is frequently associated with spasm (see Chapter 4).
- Utilise pre-emptive antispasmodic medications and vasodilators.
- Apply gentle smaller diameter catheter techniques to diminish spasm risk.
- Use BAT or CAT techniques.

3.8.2 Access Site Bleeding

To prevent and manage bleeding,

- Maintain close monitoring of the access site to ensure timely intervention if bleeding occurs;
- Meta-analyses affirm the effectiveness of RAO devices and compression techniques in reducing bleeding complications [15].

3.8.3 Haematoma Formation

Haematoma formation can cause pain and delayed ambulation. Strategies to prevent and manage haematoma involve

- Application of appropriate pressure post-procedure to prevent haematoma;
- Timely recognition and intervention, including drainage or compression if a haematoma forms; and
- If a large forearm haematoma occurs due to RA perforation, seek advice from vascular surgery and preferably manage with fingertip pressure rather than bandages and devices.

3.9 CONCLUSIONS

Having performed >7,000 TRA PCI, my personal approach (Peter O'Kane) to TRA is upfront sedation with a benzodiazepine, minimal infiltration of the RA site with lidocaine to preserve anatomy, careful single-wall RA puncture with a 21 G needle using fingertip palpation and use of a slender 6F Glidesheath. In the absence of first pass or prolonged time to access RA, I use integrated US guidance. For small radial arteries or if any resistance is encountered, I have a low threshold to visualise early with angiography and use an 0.014″ guidewire and 4F or 5F catheters to access the aorta to permit catheter exchange. I do not routinely use IA vasodilators. I adopt a "fail fast, switch quick approach" and will move to the other RA site if initially unsuccessful or consider the distal radial approach discussed in Chapter 10.

REFERENCES

1. Allen E, Edgar V. Thromboangiitis Obliterans: Methods of Diagnosis of Chronic Occlusive Arterial Lesions Distal to the Wrist With Illustrative Cases. *Amer J Med Sci.* 1929;*178*:237.

2. Ejrup B, Fischer B, Wright IS. Clinical Evaluation of Blood Flow to the Hand. The False-Positive Allen Test. *Circulation.* 1966;*33*:778–80.

3. Barbeau GR, Arsenault F, Dugas L, Simard S, Lariviere MM. Evaluation of the Ulnopalmar Arterial Arches With Pulse Oximetry and Plethysmography: Comparison With the Allen's Test in 1010 Patients. *Am Heart J.* 2004;*147*:489–93.

4. Valgimigli M, Campo G, Penzo C, et al. RADAR Investigators. Transradial Coronary Catheterization and Intervention Across the Whole Spectrum of Allen Test Results. *J Am Coll Cardiol.* 2014;*63*:1833–41. doi: 10.1016/j.jacc.2013.12.043

5. Deftereos S, Giannopoulos G, Raisakis K, Hahalis G, Kaoukis A, Kossyvakis C, Avramides D, Pappas L, Panagopoulou V, Pyrgakis V, Alexopoulos D, Stefanadis C, Cleman MW. Moderate Procedural Sedation and Opioid Analgesia During Transradial Coronary Interventions to Prevent Spasm: A Prospective Randomized Study. *JACC Cardiovasc Interv.* 2013;*6*:267–73. doi: 10.1016/j.jcin.2012.11.005

6. Youn YJ, Kim WT, Lee JW, Ahn SG, Ahn MS, Kim JY, Yoo BS, Lee SH, Yoon J, Choe KH. Eutectic Mixture of Local Anesthesia Cream Can Reduce Both the Radial Pain and Sympathetic Response During Transradial Coronary Angiography. *Korean Circ J.* 2011;*41*:726–32. doi: 10.4070/kcj.2011.41.12.726

7. Kwok CS, Rashid M, Fraser D, Nolan J, Mamas M. Intra-Arterial Vasodilators to Prevent Radial Artery Spasm: A Systematic Review and Pooled Analysis of Clinical Studies. *Cardiovasc Revasc Med.* 2015;*16*:484–90. doi: 10.1016/j.carrev.2015.08.008

8. Pancholy SB, Sanghvi KA, Patel TM. Radial Artery Access Technique Evaluation Trial: Randomized Comparison of Seldinger versus Modified Seldinger Technique for Arterial Access for Transradial Catheterization. *Catheter Cardiovasc Interv.* 2012;*80*:288–91. doi: 10.1002/ccd.23445

9. Rothschild JM. Ultrasound Guidance of Central Venous Catheterization. Making Health Care Safer: A Critical Analysis of Patient Safety Practices, Agency for Healthcare Research and Quality (2001) Evidence Report/Technology Assessment, No. 43. AHRQ Publication No. 01-E058. Rockville, MD: Agency for Healthcare Research and Quality, 2001:245–53.

10. Seto AH, Abu-Fadel MS, Sparling JM, et al. Real-Time Ultrasound Guidance Facilitates Femoral Arterial Access and Reduces Vascular Complications: FAUST (Femoral Arterial Access With Ultrasound Trial). *J Am Coll Cardiol Intv* 2010;*3*:751–8.

11. Seto AH, Roberts JS, Abu-Fadel MS, Czak SJ, Latif F, Jain SP, Raza JA, Mangla A, Panagopoulos G, Patel PM, Kern MJ, Lasic Z. Real-Time Ultrasound Guidance Facilitates Transradial Access: RAUST (Radial Artery access With Ultrasound Trial). *JACC Cardiovasc Interv.* 2015;*8*:283–91. doi: 10.1016/j.jcin.2014.05.036

12. Child N, Fernandez JP, O'Kane P Radial artery sheath reaction treated with oral steroids. *BMJ* 2011;*342*:d1287.
13. Saito S, Ikei H, Hosokawa G, Tanaka S Influence of the Ratio Between Radial Artery Inner Diameter and Sheath Outer Diameter on Radial Artery Flow After Transradial Coronary Intervention. *Catheter Cardiovasc Interv.* 1999;*46*:173–8.
14. Rathore S, Stables RH, Pauriah M, Hakeem A, Mills JD, Palmer ND, Perry RA, Morris JL. Impact of Length and Hydrophilic Coating of the Introducer Sheath on Radial Artery Spasm During Transradial Coronary Intervention: A Randomized Study. *JACC Cardiovasc Interv.* 2010;*3*:475–83. doi: 10.1016/j.jcin.2010.03.009
15. Shroff AR et al. SCAI Expert Consensus Statement Update on Best Practices for Transradial Angiography and Intervention. *Catheter Cardiovasc Interv.* 2020;*95*:245–52.

Accessing The Aorta

4

Techniques to Navigate from The Puncture Site to the Heart

Shazia T. Hussain and Shrilla Banerjee

4.1 INTRODUCTION

This chapter considers the techniques required to navigate equipment from the radial access site at the wrist into the aorta. The relevant arterial anatomy is reviewed, including common anomalies and anatomical variations which may hinder success. Techniques to aid success, including the use of upper limb angiography for procedural planning, are discussed. Strategies to deal with these challenges, including catheter and balloon-assisted tracking and the use of specific wire strategies, are described. The presence of anatomical challenges is associated with an increased risk of procedural failure. Whilst it is almost always possible to successfully complete these complex procedures, considerable skill and expertise are required, and less experienced operators

DOI: 10.1201/9781003153627-4

should seek assistance from expert colleagues to reduce the risk of iatrogenic complications.

4.2 UPPER LIMB ARTERIAL ANATOMY AND RADIAL ACCESS

Accessing the aorta from the forearm is a superior access route with proven mortality benefits and fewer access site complications for patients, but it requires specific training and expertise for the operator [1, 2]. The right brachiocephalic artery branches from the proximal aorta and gives rise to the right subclavian artery (the left subclavian artery arises directly from the more distal aortic arch), which enters the upper limb as the axillary then brachial artery. The radial artery is a continuation of the brachial artery as it divides into the ulnar and radial artery at the antecubital fossa. The radial artery runs on the lateral aspect of the arm. It extends to the styloid process of the anterior surface of the radius and runs across the floor of the anatomical snuffbox to the palm of the hand, where it provides palmar and dorsal carpal branches creating the palmar and dorsal carpal arches which anastomose with the branches of the ulnar artery and provide an extensive system of collateral blood supply which protects the hand from ischaemia in most circumstances. Figure 4.1 shows the anatomical landmarks and access points for the standard radial and ulnar punctures.

4.3 USE OF UPPER LIMB ANGIOGRAPHY TO GUIDE ACCESS TO THE AORTA

Catheter laboratory set-up and puncture access technique are described in Chapters 2 and 3.

The radial sheath pack usually includes a 0.018 to 0.021-inch short wire to allow initial radial access. This has a soft tip but is a stiff wire, so it does not have the trackability to traverse the radial artery but has enough stiffness to allow passage of the dilator and sheath.

After successful placement of the radial access sheath, best practice suggests taking a forearm angiogram [3, 4]. This allows the identification of anatomical variants (high radial bifurcations, loops, and tortuosity are the most

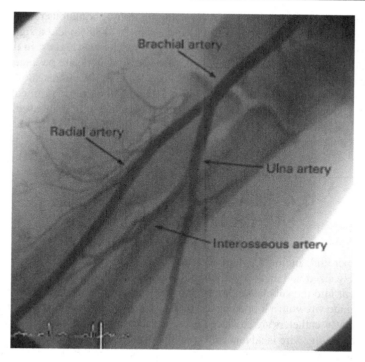

FIGURE 4.1 Arm angiogram demonstrating normal anatomy.

frequent anomalous findings) that might make the passage of the access wire more difficult. The angiogram is obtained with the arm positioned so that the patient's palm faces the laboratory ceiling, rotating enough to separate the bony landmarks of the radial head ulnar olecranon on X-ray screening. This separates the vessels so that they are optimally visualised without vascular overlap, facilitating analysis of the anatomical situation. Injection of contrast into the forearm arteries can cause short-lived discomfort for the patient, and it is important to warn them of this in advance of the angiography. A syringe containing 5 ml of contrast is attached to the radial sheath side arm and mixed with aspirated blood – this minimises angiography-related arm discomfort. The image intensifier is positioned over the forearm, and a stored fluoroscopy image is obtained during contrast injection. A single injection will normally display arterial anatomy from the tip of the radial sheath to the upper brachial artery and be sufficient to allow procedural planning. In unusual or complex anatomical situations, additional angulated or more proximal views may be required.

In a study assessing routine forearm angiography, anomalous radial artery anatomy was demonstrated to be relatively common (13.8%) and a significant cause of procedural failure. The procedural failure rate was highest in patients with radial loops (37.1%). As there are methods by which safe passage of the wire and catheters can be achieved, prior knowledge of anomalies should help avoid complications or procedural failure [5]. In challenging anatomical situations, additional vasodilator, analgesia, and sedation agents can be used proactively to minimise discomfort. Consideration of bilateral/universal catheters to reduce the number of exchanges may also be helpful (see Section 5.4.3).

4.4 MANAGING NORMAL UPPER LIMB ARTERIES

If the upper limb angiogram demonstrates that the radial and brachial arteries are adequately sized and anatomy is normal (Figure 4.1), the passage of wires and equipment into the subclavian artery is usually straightforward. A conventional 0.035″ guidewire with a looped tip can usually be easily passed into the aorta, and subsequently, catheters are advanced over the access wire with minimal technical difficulty. As the wire is advanced, screening can begin at the patient's shoulder level, and the wire should be visualised as it passes through the subclavian artery and into the aorta, minimising radiation exposure. Difficulty traversing important subclavian tortuosity is discussed later in this chapter. In such normal anatomy, the only common problem is radial spasm (Figure 4.2). If spasm is encountered, we recommend the administration of vasodilators, analgesia, and light sedation. The angiogram can then be repeated to assess response. If the spasm resolves, a 0.035″ hydrophilic small J-tipped wire (such as a Terumo Baby J wire) could be used in combination with catheter-assisted tracking (CAT – described later in this chapter and in Chapter 7) to minimise the risk of inducing further spasm. Consideration of downsizing from 6F to 5F and the use of universal catheters to minimise exchanges is also recommended.

4.5 MANAGING ANOMALOUS UPPER LIMB ARTERIES

Radial artery anomalies are frequently encountered. The most common radial abnormality is a high bifurcating radial artery (Figure 4.3), which arises from the brachial artery above the antecubital fossa (present in around 15%

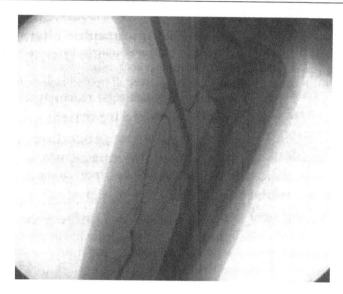

FIGURE 4.2   Long segment of severe spasm in proximal portion of radial artery.

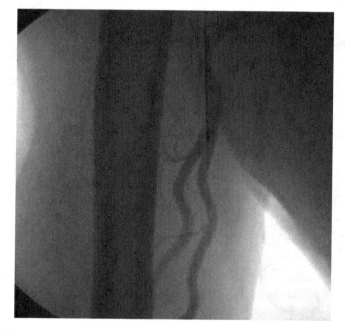

FIGURE 4.3   Large-diameter high bifurcation of radial artery arising above the elbow joint from mid brachial artery.

of individuals). Many of these high bifurcating vessels are of small diameter and therefore prone to spasm. This spasm can be severe and result in catheter entrapment. If the upper limb angiogram demonstrates a large-diameter high bifurcating vessel, there are usually no technical difficulties. If the vessel is small in diameter, then downsizing of equipment; upfront liberal use of vasodilator, analgesic, and sedation medications; and the use of universal diagnostic or guiding catheters to reduce the need for catheter exchanges will minimise the spasm risk.

Radial loops (Figure 4.4) are a common cause for failure of radial access and the frequency of these has been reported as 2%–3% [5]. Many loops are accompanied by a small-diameter recurrent radial artery at the apex of the loop, which assumes a straight path into the upper arm. The presence of this branch has the potential to complicate the procedure if angiography hasn't been performed. In the presence of an unsuspected loop, a wire may advance via the loop and into the recurrent artery in the upper arm. The position of the wire may replicate that of a normally tracking wire in the brachial artery.

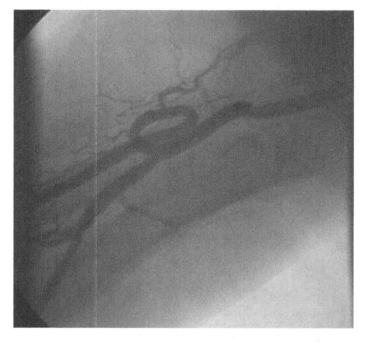

FIGURE 4.4 Large-diameter radial loop.

Equipment advanced into this small vessel will frequently cause dissection or perforation, leading to procedural failure.

Most loops can be straightened, but when they are of large diameter, this is usually accompanied by a significant amount of rotational force within the straightened arterial segment, leading to severe spasm. If the arm angiogram demonstrates the presence of a large-diameter radial loop, it may be preferable to look for an alternative access site. Smaller-diameter loops are less challenging, but a standard 0.035″ wire often fails to traverse even these small-diameter loops due to friction effects. We recommend using a highly trackable 0.035″ hydrophilic coated wire that will traverse the loop without excessive friction. It is important to choose a wire with a looped tip (such as the Terumo Baby J wire), as this configuration will reliably track within the lumen. Hydrophilic wires with angulated tips have an increased propensity to track into side branches or pass easily through angulated vessel walls, causing perforation and procedural failure. When the wire has been advanced into the proximal vasculature, gentle traction will often straighten the loop. Catheters should then be tracked through the straightened loop with the aid of CAT to minimise the risk of spasm induction. If the 0.035″ hydrophilic J-tipped wire fails to traverse the loop, a 0.014″ interventional wire combined with balloon-assisted tracking (BAT – described later in this chapter and in Chapter 7) will often succeed [6–8].

Other forearm anatomical anomalies can occur. Extreme radial tortuosity can be overcome with the use of hydrophilic or interventional wires combined with CAT or BAT. Rarer radial anomalies include hypoplasia, complex bifurcation anatomy, and radial artery stenosis, for which alternative access should be sought.

4.6 TRAVERSING THE BRACHIAL AND SUBCLAVIAN ARTERIES

In contrast to the radial artery, loops and anomalies in the brachial artery are relatively infrequent. In a normal straight brachial artery, the passage of wires and equipment is usually simple and low risk. A 360° brachial loop may be encountered, particularly in older individuals. Although they can be managed as described for radial loops (see Section 4.5), great care is needed, as iatrogenic trauma to the brachial artery may lead to major ischaemia in the forearm. Operators early in their learning curve should always seek advice and guidance from an experienced operator before attempting to straighten a brachial loop.

Subclavian, innominate, and aortic arch anatomical challenges include tortuosity, loops, stenosis, and congenital aberrancy [9]. Subclavian tortuosity

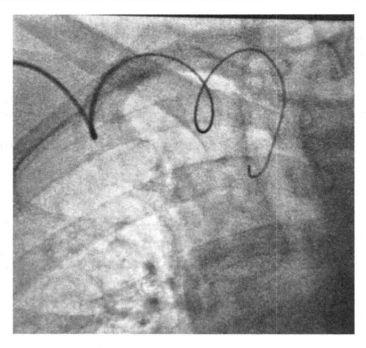

FIGURE 4.5   Extreme subclavian tortuosity.

(Figure 4.5) is more common on the right side and in older individuals. Consequently, some operators preferentially choose left radial access in patients over 85 years of age to minimise technical complexity and consequent procedural failure rates. Tortuosity is particularly common at the innominate-aortic junction. Additionally, in older hypertensive patients, the upper aorta is often distorted or elongated, as vessels tend to respond to hypertension by becoming more circuitous. This can prove difficult to navigate, but once again, fluoroscopic capture of an angiogram can make the situation clearer and facilitate navigation. The most frequent technically challenging congenital anomaly is the occurrence of a retro-oesophageal subclavian (prevalence is around 1 in 400). In this situation, the right subclavian takes an aberrant course, crossing the midline and joining the distal aortic arch (Figure 4.6). It should be suspected when the access wire or catheters track far to the left side of the mediastinum before taking a tortuous course and retrograde passage to the aortic root. Coronary procedures are possible in these circumstances but can be very technically challenging and should only be attempted if the access options are limited and the operator is highly experienced – in most circumstances, it is preferable to switch the access site.

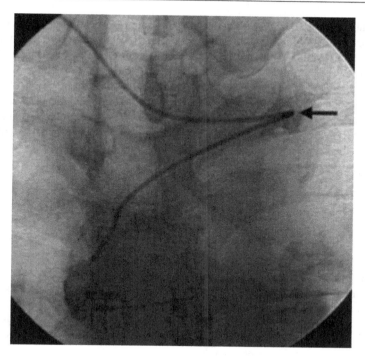

FIGURE 4.6 Retro-oesophageal subclavian – catheter tracking across midline to enter aorta in distal position before tracking back to cross midline and enter ascending aorta.

In many cases of subclavian tortuosity, asking the patient to inhale deeply can assist the passage of a standard 0.035″ wire, as this action pulls down the diaphragm, extending the aorta and potentially straightening out areas of tortuosity. If this manoeuvre fails, the 0.035″ wire can be replaced by a hydrophilic wire with a looped tip (e.g., Terumo Baby J wire) that will traverse the curves and loops and eventually pass into the ascending aorta and down to the coronary ostia. With gentle but sustained pressure, the loops will often straighten, and the wire will successfully traverse the artery. Using a 0.014″ interventional wire may also help, especially when used in conjunction with the BAT technique.

In cases of subclavian/innominate artery tortuosity, crossing the tortuous segment is not the only technical difficulty. Once catheters have accessed the aorta, it may require considerable manipulation to cannulate the coronaries with an attendant risk of catheter kinking or compromised catheter performance. This can be managed by attaching an angioplasty O-ring connector to the catheter to facilitate leaving a 0.035″ wire in the catheter lumen whilst torquing the catheter into place to avoid kinking whilst manipulating. If satisfactory coronary intubation is not possible, an alternative access site is required. In cases of challenging anatomy, we recommend exchanging catheters over a long exchange wire, as this maintains wire access to the aorta and limits the need to recross with each exchange. Occasionally, the catheters follow the wrong path and pass into the descending aorta. In this case, an angiogram may help, but also passing the catheter to the level of the arch and then directing the wire and then the catheter towards the right-hand side of the patient will frequently allow access.

4.7 BALLOON-ASSISTED AND CATHETER-ASSISTED TRACKING

In situations of extreme spasm or challenging anatomy, BAT or CAT is recommended (Figure 4.1). These techniques overcome the razor effect (Figure 4.4) of the sharp guide catheter edge contacting the arterial wall, which may provoke further spasm[10]. The BAT technique can be used to facilitate the delivery of 5F or 6F diagnostic or guiding catheters when an angioplasty wire has been used to traverse challenging anatomy. The CAT technique is used to deliver guiding catheters when a 0.035″ wire is positioned in the aorta. These techniques are described in more detail in Chapter 7.

4.8 CONCLUSIONS

Performing an initial upper limb angiogram after placement of the radial access sheath is an important way to identify potential procedural difficulties and plan an optimal procedure. In many patients with satisfactory anatomy, there are few technical challenges. In the presence of upper limb vascular challenge there are strategies that can be employed to facilitate procedural success. These should be employed with caution. During an operator's learning curve, a challenging anatomical situation should prompt the operator to seek help from an experienced colleague. In some circumstances, upper limb anatomical complexity may preclude access from the radial artery.

REFERENCES

1. Gargiulo et al. Effects on Mortality and Major Bleeding of Radial Versus Femoral Artery Access for Coronary Angiography or Percutaneous Coronary Intervention: Meta-Analysis of Individual Patient Data From 7 Multicenter Randomized Clinical Trials. *Circulation.* 2022;*146*:1329–43.
2. Alnasser SM et al. Transradial Approach for Coronary Angiography and Intervention in the Elderly: A Meta-Analysis of 777,841 Patients. *Int J Cardiol.* 2017;*228*:45–51.
3. Biljana Z et al. Benefits of Routine Preprocedural Radial Artery Angiography in STEMI Patients. *Cath Cardiovasc Int.* 2019;*93*:25–31.
4. Kern M et al. Use of Radiobrackial Angiography in Transradial Cardiac Catheterisation and Intervention. *Cardiovasc Revasc Med.* 2020;*21*:797–803.
5. Lo TS et al. Radial Artery Anomaly and Its Influence on Transradial Coronary Procedural Outcome. *Heart.* 2008;*95*:410–15.
6. Patel T, Shah S, Pancholy S. Balloon-Assisted Tracking of a Guide Catheter Through Difficult Radial Anatomy: A Technical Report. *Catheter Cardiovasc Interv.* 2013;*81*:E215–18.
7. Garg N, Sahoo D, Goel PK. Pigtail Assisted Tracking of Guide Catheter for Navigating the Difficult Radial: Overcoming the "Razor Effect". *Indian Heart J* 2016;*68*:355–60.
8. Scoccia A et al. Mother-in-Child Assisted Tracking (MiCAT): A Mechanical Technique to Overcome Severe Radial Artery Spasm. *J Invasive Cardiol* 2022;*34*:E588–93.
9. Patel T et al. Working Through Challenges of Subclavian, Innominate, and Aortic Arch Regions During Transradial Approach. *Catheter Cardiovasc Interv* 2014;*84*:224–35.

Catheter Selection and Image Acquisition

5

Afzal Hayat and Azfar Zaman

5.1 INTRODUCTION

Transradial access (TRA) is well established and endorsed as the preferred route of access for coronary diagnostic and interventional procedures [1, 2]. This change has been driven by consistent data showing TRA is associated with reduced risk of access site bleeding, vascular complications, and reduced mortality in patients with acute coronary syndromes (ACS) compared to transfemoral access [3–7]. Using the distal radial artery in the anatomical snuffbox (see Chapter 10) has potential advantages compared to the traditional approach from the proximal radial artery – catheter options for this approach are similar to those for the conventional proximal radial approach [8]. Transradial cases can be performed without any compromise to procedural quality and outcome – this requires the selection of optimal catheter configurations to ensure atraumatic coaxial coronary intubation. Catheter selection options are different than those for femoral procedures. This chapter will provide recommendations for choosing the optimal catheters in radial access cases.

DOI: 10.1201/9781003153627-5

5.2 CATHETER DESIGN FEATURES

Catheters can be classified into diagnostic and guide catheters. Diagnostic catheters have thicker shafts, tapering soft tips, smaller internal diameter, and a strong, thick, two-layer wall construction. These features confer good catheter kink resistance and torque response and permit high injection pressures. The internal lumen is too small to allow delivery of coronary devices. Their design and simple structure make them robust and easy to torque, although small French gauges (e.g., 4F diagnostics) can occasionally be too pliable to provide a reliable 1:1 response. Guide catheters have thinner walls, stiffer shafts, non-tapered tips, larger lumens, and reinforced construction with three layers (Figure 5.1) [9]. The outer nylon elastomer layer offers a low-friction atraumatic surface. Structural strength derives from stainless steel braiding. The inner PTFE (Teflon) layer is a highly lubricious material that permits the passage of guidewires, balloons, and stents without obstruction. Guide catheters have differential stiffness along their lengths, with the stiffest part being near the hub that gradually transitions to the most distal, softer tip to prevent vascular injury. Thin-walled guide catheters have larger lumens than similar diagnostic catheters to facilitate the passage of equipment.

Advances in catheter design and engineering have made engagement from the radial access effective and safe. Several characteristics integrate to allow operators consistent and safe procedural success, including torque control, pushability, flexibility, kink resistance, radio-opacity, and an atraumatic tip. Operators need to be aware of the characteristics of individual catheters and will develop preferences over time. For radial operators, an understanding of the vascular anatomy, good technique with careful catheter manipulation, and awareness of pressure waveforms to avoid catheter tip damping are crucial in

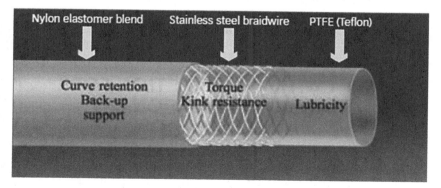

FIGURE 5.1   The three layers of a guide catheter.

preventing complications. Vascular catheters are designed to be lubricious with smooth surfaces that permit atraumatic passage through vascular conduits [10]. A randomised study from a high-volume UK centre demonstrated that lubricity and hydrophilicity were more important than the use of long radial sheaths in preventing radial spasm [11]. Enhanced lubricity reduced vascular spasm and enabled negotiation of calcified branch vessels, particularly at the innominate, across the aortic arch, and in the left subclavian [12]. The Asahi system of Eaucaths has been demonstrated to overcome resistant radial spasm in a prospective observational study [13].

Catheters come in different sizes, shapes, and lengths (typically 90–110 cm). Longer catheters of up to 125 cm are necessary for tortuous anatomy or when negotiating gross dilatation of the aortic root and ascending aorta. Long 125 cm catheters (pigtail or multipurpose) are helpful when interrogating abdominal or iliac vessels – e.g., during vascular intervention undertaken from the upper limb. This may be necessary for minimal access trans-catheter aortic valve intervention (TAVI), where radial access is used to introduce balloons to control lower limb peripheral access site bleeding. Commonly used catheters for TRA for standard anatomy are discussed in this section. The list is not exhaustive, and significant variation in anatomy may call for unusual catheter choices. Increasing experience with a variety of catheters will increase confidence and familiarity when tackling unusual coronary anatomies.

The external diameter of catheters is determined using the French catheter scale with 1F approximating 0.33 mm. The external diameter of a 6F diagnostic and guide catheter is thus equal to 2 mm. The internal diameter of a 6F diagnostic catheter is 1.4 mm. Due to their different construction guide, catheters have larger internal diameters than diagnostic catheters (the internal diameter of 6F guide catheter (GC) is typically 1.8 mm). The most commonly used diagnostic catheters in adults are 5F–6F. GCs are typically 6F–8F. In general, larger calibre guide catheters are reserved for more complex percutaneous coronary intervention (PCI), where multiple wires, bulky equipment, and simultaneous balloons or stents may be required. As a general principle, smaller-diameter catheters are preferred for radial cases to minimise access site injury.

5.3 CATHETER SELECTION FOR TRANSRADIAL CORONARY ANGIOGRAPHY

This is influenced by several factors, including procedure access site (classical radial, distal radial, left or right access), height and weight of the patient, aortic size/configuration, angulation of coronaries, operator experience, and presence of grafts. Coronary ostium location may be high, low, anterior, posterior, or anomalous. Coronary take-offs may be superior, horizontal, inferior, or Shepherd's crook right coronary artery (RCA only). Coaxial engagement of coronary ostia is key to achieving safe engagement and opacification during angiography, and this is achieved through the selection of the appropriate catheter configuration. There are a wide range of catheter configurations available.

Judkins catheters were originally designed for the femoral route. They are pre-shaped catheters with a primary and secondary curve designed such that little manipulation is required if used from the femoral artery. They have a standard length of 100 cm and a range of sizes determined by the length of the catheter between primary and secondary curves ranging from 3.5 to 6. Although designed for transfemoral access, they are suitable for transradial angiography and some PCI cases.

Amplatz right (AR) and Amplatz left (AL) catheters come in multiple sizes with increasing curvature. Amplatz catheters are more suitable for abnormal coronary ostia, such as high and posterior LM origin, separate origins of LAD and LCx, high anterior RCA, or Shepherd's Crook RCA. Whilst engaging with Amplatz catheters, it is essential to note that pulling on the catheter will cause deep engagement, increasing dissection risk. Similarly, an AR shape can engage right coronaries with an abnormally high anterior or inferior origin. However, the primary curve and distal tip length of the AR are relatively short, making stable guide support less effective in practice.

The multipurpose (MP) catheter was initially used as a single universal catheter for brachial procedures. This is a polyurethane catheter with a simple curve, a straight tip, and an end hole plus side holes. The MP catheter can be used for both right and left coronary angiography, ventriculography, right-sided grafts, and right heart catheterisation. Its use for cardiac catheterisation requires careful manipulation within the aortic root, and it is therefore not suitable for inexperienced operators. There are also specific radial universal catheters that are designed to facilitate angiography of both coronaries with a single catheter (see Section 5.4.3).

5.4 CORONARY CANNULATION

5.4.1 Left Coronary Intubation

The native left coronary artery can be engaged in the majority of patients by using a Judkins left 3.5 (JL3.5). From the right radial, and to some extent the left radial, the JL catheter is elongated by the bend in the innominate artery and made to point downward, hence the need to use the smaller JL 3.5. The left coronary ostium can be engaged at 30° to 45° in left anterior oblique (LAO) or posteroanterior (PA) views. For less experienced operators or in cases of challenging engagement, the LAO view is preferred as the plane of coronary ostia is orthogonal to the line of sight in this view, and the ascending aorta and sinus of Valsalva are not superimposed on coronary ostia optimising visualisation. Experienced operators often use a PA projection for intubation of the left coronary, as it reduces backscatter radiation exposure. The JL is advanced into the aortic root over a wire and rotated towards the left main coronary ostium. After slow wire removal, the catheter is connected to the pressure monitoring system, and having confirmed a good aortic pressure, trace contrast is injected gently to establish position. Gentle rotational movements, combined with slow withdrawal or advancement of the catheter, will usually engage the left coronary. If the JL3.5 fails through folding up, then changing to a JL4 is often sufficient. In the presence of an anomalous anatomical situation, Amplatz, multipurpose, or dedicated radial curves will usually solve the issue.

5.4.2 Right Coronary Intubation

For the native right coronary, most can be engaged using the standard JR4 catheter. In the LAO view, the catheter is advanced into the aortic root, and rotation combined with a gentle withdrawal or advancement will guide the catheter to the ostium. In anomalous anatomical situations, an Amplatz or MP will often succeed.

5.4.3 Universal Catheters for Transradial Coronary Angiography

There are dedicated transradial catheters designed to allow imaging of both the right and left coronaries with a single catheter. The benefit of using a single catheter for both coronaries is the minimisation of catheter exchange with a reduced risk of radial artery spasm. However, achieving coaxial engagement can be challenging, leading to suboptimal imaging. There is a risk of deep engagement with inferior take-offs, and selective conus cannulation is greater with inferior take-off RCAs; consequently, universal catheters need careful handling to prevent these issues.

The Tiger family of dedicated radial catheters have a curve design configured to facilitate cannulation of both coronary ostia. The tip of the Tiger catheter points up, whereas that of the Jacky points down. They come in 5 and 6 Fr sizes. A side hole in the tip of the Tiger may reduce the risk of intimal injury during injection in non-coaxial engagement but results in greater contrast use. Tiger catheters are available in two modified configurations (Tiger 1 and Tiger 2) and have demonstrated good performance for transradial angiography with a useful reduction in the occurrence of radial spasm in randomised trials.

The Tiger is deployed into the ascending aorta, and pressure monitoring is established. The catheter is then advanced and rotated and will usually easily canulate both coronary ostia. Tiger catheter has a learning curve related to difficulty in cannulating both ostia and deep intubation of the right coronary. During the learning curve phase, it is appropriate to have a low threshold to switch to a Judkins catheter if bilateral coronary intubation is difficult. The DxTerity catheter is an alternative universal radial diagnostic catheter that also has data that supports its use for reducing procedure duration [14].

5.4.4 Vein Graft Angiography

Saphenous vein bypass grafts are usually placed on the anterior surface of the ascending aorta – the RCA grafts are on the right anterior surface, and the LCA grafts are on the left anterior surface. The LCA grafts can be canulated in the RAO or LAO view. The RCA grafts are usually canulated in the LAO view. A JR4 can be used as the first catheter to look for grafts. If this fails, an multipurpose angiography (MPA) or right coronary bypass (RCB) shape can be used for right coronary grafts and an AL1 for left coronary grafts. Some operators prefer to switch to an AL shape immediately, using this for cannulation of the native right and for saphenous grafts, obviating the need for further catheter changes [15]. If these catheters fail, a left coronary bypass (LCB) catheter can be beneficial, although it may not have sufficient reach to access the origin of left-sided grafts when approaching from the right radial. In experienced hands, the Tiger 1 catheter can be used from the left radial to access both the native vessels and vein grafts, though it is often more difficult to opacify the RCA grafts due to their downward course, which may require switching to an MPA. Nevertheless, using a Tiger first can minimise exchanges and identify the origin of most grafts, including the left internal mammary (LIMA), and may assist in decision-making prior to exchanging to an alternative catheter if required.

5.4.5 Internal Mammary Graft Angiography

A large proportion of patients have a combination of venous grafts and a single LIMA arterial graft, which originates from the left subclavian artery. The left radial approach is preferable in these patients, as it facilitates cannulation of the LIMA graft, vein grafts, and native coronaries via a single arterial puncture.

A JR4 is often used to image the native RCA and possible vein grafts. As the JR4 is withdrawn into the subclavian, gentle rotation and contrast administration will often identify the LIMA origin, allowing cannulation with the JR4. If this fails, a specific internal mammary (IM) catheter may be necessary. The IM catheter resembles a JR4 but with a tighter primary curve (80°) and a longer tip. It is usually simple to engage the LIMA with an IM catheter from the left radial over a 0.035" wire passed to the ascending aorta. Cautious withdrawal of the catheter distally along the left subclavian with careful test injection allows identification and then selective cannulation of the LIMA. If the JR4 and LIMA catheters fail, the Bartorelli-Cozzi is another dedicated LIMA catheter that may be successful.

If the patient has bilateral mammary arterial grafts, there are a number of options. A femoral approach allows both subclavian arteries to be cannulated from a single access site for bilateral mammary graft imaging. A simultaneous left and right radial approach is a simple solution if femoral access is unfavourable. For expert operators, both subclavian vessels can be accessed from the right radial access site. The RIMA is imaged in a conventional manner. A Simmons or Judkins left catheter is then advanced through the right subclavian into the aorta, rotated and positioned close to the origin of the contralateral subclavian artery. Gentle rotation and contrast injection will usually identify the origin of this vessel. A 0.035" guidewire is advanced into the vessel to facilitate catheter deployment into the contralateral subclavian and LIMA imaging. This is a complex and demanding technique, with a risk of vascular injury, and should only be attempted by expert operators.

5.5 GUIDE CATHETER SELECTION

The selection of an optimal GC configuration for coronary intervention depends on several factors, including the following:

- Size of ascending aorta
- Target vessel calibre
- Orientation of ostium
- Tortuosity and calcification of target vessel
- Complexity of procedure (e.g., bifurcation stenting requiring kissing balloon inflation, heavily calcified lesions requiring the use of atherectomy devices)

An ideal GC should provide adequate backup support during the procedure whilst minimising the risk of vascular injury. Catheters should facilitate coaxial and stable engagement. Various dedicated radial catheters have been introduced, but the standard shapes remain the mainstay of coronary intervention for many operators.

Passive support is provided by guide design and its ability to sit against the opposite aortic wall (Figures 5.2 and 5.3). Active support is achieved by manipulating the guide into the coronary vessel, enabling deep engagement. Larger catheters (such as 7 or 8 Fr) provide better passive support but are difficult to manipulate. Smaller catheters (5 or 6 Fr) are easier to manipulate and achieve deep engagement if required. Some shapes are better at providing passive support but can't be easily manipulated, such as Amplatz catheters.

Many PCI procedures can be performed with 6F catheters. If staged stent deployment is used, two-stent bifurcation PCI can be performed without recourse to larger guides. Simultaneous balloons can be deployed within 6F GCs, but the maximal inner diameter should be checked to ensure compatibility, as it does vary between manufacturers. Escalation to more complex technology or the use of simultaneous device deployment will usually require upgrading to a 7F GC. For rotational atherectomy (rotablation), it is important to match GC and burr size (see Table 5.1). This will avoid contact between the burr and catheter wall within the system and reduce the risk of catheter material being micro-embolised during burr rotation.

TABLE 5.1 Rotablator GC compatibility

	BURR (MM)	DIAMETER (INCHES)	MINIMUM RECOMMENDED GUIDE CATHETER INTERNAL DIAMETER (INCHES)	RECOMMENDED GUIDE CATHETER SIZE (FRENCH)[a]
Guide sizes are	1.25	0.049	0.060[b]	6.0
based on larger	1.50	0.059	0.063	6.0
lumen catheters	1.75	0.069	0.073	7.0
	2.00	0.079	0.083	8.0
	2.15	0.085	0.089	8.0
	2.25	0.089	0.093	9.0
	2.38	0.094	0.098	9.0
	2.50	0.098	0.102	10.0

Notes
[a] Inside guide catheter diameter and french size may differ among manufacturers.
[b] Ensure guide is compatible with the largest burr intended to be used.

5.5.1 Guide Selection for Left Coronary Artery Intervention

For most left coronary interventional procedures EBU/XB catheters in the size range of 3.5–5 provide excellent backup due to their apposition to the opposite aortic wall or sinus (Figure 5.2). It is important to size the guide appropriately to maximise support. Frequently, larger curve sizes are required when approaching from the radial route, such as using an EBU 3.75 or 4, in place of the more commonly used 3.5.

Due to their unfavourable configuration, JL catheters were not designed principally to provide backup support during PCI and are inadequate for many PCIs. This feature can be advantageous for selected cases of ostial left main lesions when cannulation depth needs to be restricted. When ostial anatomy is anomalous, Amplatz or dedicated radial guides may be needed.

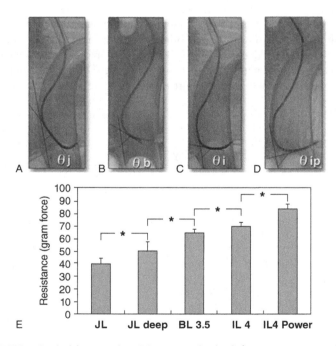

FIGURE 5.2   Optimising passive GC support in the left coronary artery from the radial approach. The top panel shows catheters deployed in a model of the aorta and left coronary artery. The bottom panel displays the resistance to catheter displacement of the different configurations. Moving from A (judkins configuration) to D (IKARI) is associated with increased support as this configuration is well applied to the contralateral aortic wall.

5.5.2 Guide Selection for Right Coronary Intervention

Judkins right catheters (usually a JR4) can be used for most PCI cases (Figure 5.3). However, they provide poor backup support during complex PCI or in a patient with a dilated aorta. In these cases, buddy wires, extra support wires or deep intubation techniques may be required to successfully complete the procedure. As an alternative to deep intubation of the GC, the use of guide extension catheters facilitates the use of a standard Judkins right catheter with greater confidence in challenging anatomy. For more complex procedures, catheter shapes that provide better intrinsic support include the AR (1 or 2) or AL (0.75, 1 or 2). A cautious approach with Amplatz catheters is required to reduce the risk of coronary dissection. The latter can occur with failure to control deep intubation and with the use of catheters with rigid tips.

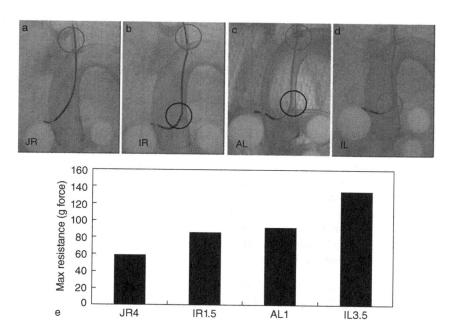

FIGURE 5.3 Optimising passive guide catheter support in the RCA from the radial approach. The top panel shows catheters deployed in a model of the aorta and RCA. The bottom panel displays the resistance to catheter displacement of the different configurations. Moving from A (JR4) to D (IKARI) is associated with increased support as this configuration is well applied to the contralateral aortic wall.

5.5.3 Dedicated Radial Guide Catheters for Right and Left Coronary PCI

The propensity of radial arteries to develop spasm with multiple GC exchanges makes the use of a single catheter appealing for the engagement of both right and left coronary arteries. The Barbeau catheter is a modified multipurpose catheter with an extra 135° curve at the tip to facilitate cannulation of both coronary ostia. The Kimney has a 45° primary curve and a secondary curve of 90° that allows it to support itself against the opposite aortic wall to optimise support. The left coronary artery can be engaged from below, and the right coronary from a horizontal or superior position. Ikari left and right catheters are designed to offer optimal support during radial PCI. With minimal modification to technique, the Ikari left can intubate the right and left coronary ostia so that interventions can be performed in both vessels with a single catheter.

Compared to Judkins, these catheters provide better backup support but have not been compared to EBU- or XB-type curves. Studies of ST elevation myocardial infarction (STEMI) patients using dedicated bilateral radial GCs demonstrate that high rates of procedural success with significant beneficial reductions in door-to-balloon time, procedure duration, and equipment usage are achievable [16–18]. These catheters all have their own learning curve, and operators will need to be skilled in their use to replicate these favourable STEMI results.

5.5.4 Guide Selection for Graft Intervention

Graft interventions are usually technically less challenging if performed from the left arm. This allows easy intervention in mammary grafts using an IM guide. Right coronary interventions can be performed with a JR4, RCB, or multipurpose guide. LAD or circumflex vein graft interventions are usually performed with Amplatz or LCB guides. Circumflex vein grafts can be difficult to cannulate, compromising GC support – adjunctive measures such as a GC extension often resolve this issue.

5.5.5 Sheathless Radial Catheters

The maximum size of the guiding catheter that can be used for TRI is limited by the relatively small lumen of the radial artery [19]. This potentially limits backup support and the types of adjunctive devices and procedures that can be performed via TRA. A further issue is radial artery injury leading to occlusion, the most frequent post-procedure complication of TRA. This is important as it prevents the use of the ipsilateral TRA for future procedures. The sheath-to-artery diameter ratio is an important predictor of radial artery occlusion, with occlusion rates increasing with large sheath sizes [19, 20]. Strategies that facilitate transradial use for complex PCI whilst maintaining radial artery patency are important. A sheathless GC can potentially facilitate the use of larger GC systems. Traditionally, an introducer sheath with an outer diameter nearly 2F larger than the corresponding guiding catheter has been used for transradial PCI. Using a guiding catheter without an introducer sheath allows the use of larger lumen guiding catheters and may reduce trauma to the radial artery. Several sheathless catheters, including the Hyperion GC (SHGC, Asahi Intecc, Aichi, Japan), are available. These catheters maximise internal diameter and guide support whilst minimising the outer diameter and radial artery trauma. They have been designed for direct insertion (with a long tapered introducer) without the need for initial sheath placement and have favourable external diameters compared to the same-size radial sheath. Techniques for sheathless introduction of conventional GCs exist and are discussed further in Chapter 7.

5.6 CONCLUSIONS

Choosing the correct coronary catheter for radial artery access is a decision that requires a thorough understanding of the patient's anatomy, available catheters, and operator experience. Radial access, whilst a safer access route than femoral, requires awareness of radial artery physiology, anatomical variations, and the appropriate use of differing catheter designs for specific purposes. Modern diagnostic and GC technology makes diagnostic and PCI cases safe and predictably successful from radial access.

REFERENCES

1. Romagnoli E, Biondi-Zoccai G, Sciahbasi A et al. Radial versus Femoral Randomized Investigation in ST-Segment Elevation Acute Coronary Syndrome: The RIFLE-STEACS (Radial versus Femoral Randomized Investigation in ST-Elevation Acute Coronary Syndrome) Study. *J Am Coll Cardiol*. 2012;60(24):2481–9.
2. Ferrante G, Rao SV, Jüni P et al. Radial versus Femoral Access for Coronary Interventions Across the Entire Spectrum of Patients With Coronary Artery Disease: A Meta-Analysis of Randomized Trials. *J Am Coll Cardiol Intv*. 2016;9(14):1419–34.

3. Neumann F-J, Sousa-Uva M, Ahlsson A et al. 2018 ESC/EACTS Guidelines on Myocardial Revascularisation. *Eur Heart J.* 2019;*40*:87–165.
4. Mason PJ, Shah B, Tamis-Holland JE et al. An Update on Radial Artery Access and Best Practices for Trans Radial Coronary Angiography and Intervention in Acute Coronary Syndrome: A Scientific Statement From the American Heart Association. *Circ Cardiovasc Interv.* 2018;*11*(9):e000035.
5. Jolly SS, Yusuf S, Cairns J et al. Radial versus Femoral Access for Coronary Angiography and Intervention in Patients With Acute Coronary Syndromes (RIVAL): A Randomised, Parallel Group, Multicentre Trial. *The Lancet.* 2011;*377* (9775):1409–20.
6. Valgimigli M, Gagnor A, Calabró P et al. Radial versus Femoral Access in Patients With Acute Coronary Syndromes Undergoing Invasive Management: A Randomised Multicentre Trial. *The Lancet.* 2015;*385*(9986):2465–76.
7. Valgimigli M, Frigoli E, Leonardi S et al. Radial versus Femoral Access and Bivalirudin versus Unfractionated Heparin in Invasively Managed Patients With Acute Coronary Syndrome (MATRIX): Final 1-Year Results of a Multicentre, Randomised Controlled Trial. *Lancet (London, England).* 2018;*392*:835–48.
8. Sgueglia GA, Di Giorgio A, Gaspardone A, Babunashvili A. Anatomic Basis and Physiological Rationale of Distal Radial Artery Access for Percutaneous Coronary and Endovascular Procedures. *JACC Cardiovasc Interv.* 2018 Oct 22;*11*(20):2113–19. doi: 10.1016/j.jcin.2018.04.045
9. Ali R, Greenbaum AB, Kugelmass AD. A Review of Available Angioplasty Guiding Catheters, Wires and Balloons – Making the Right Choice, *Interv Cardiol.* 2012;*7*(2):100–3.
10. Saito S, Tanaka S, Hiroe Y et al. The Usefulness of Hydrophilic Coating on Arterial Sheath Introducer in Trans-Radial Coronary Intervention. *Catheter Cardiovasc Interv.* 2002;*56*(3):328–33.
11. Rathore S, Stables RH, Pauriah M, Hakeem A, Mills JD, Palmer ND, Perry RA, Morris JL. Impact of Length and Hydrophilic Coating of the Introducer Sheath on Radial Artery Spasm During Trans-Radial Coronary Intervention: A Randomised Study. *JACC Cardiovasc Interv.* 2010 May;*3*(5):475–83. doi: 10.1016/j.jcin.2010.03.009
12. Barbeau GR. Radial Loop and Extreme Vessel Tortuosity in the Trans-Radial Approach: Advantage of Hydrophilic-Coated Guidewires and Catheters. *Catheter Cardiovasc Interv.* 2003 Aug;*59*(4):442–50. doi: 10.1002/ccd.10586
13. Borrie A, Raina A, Fairley S, Ranchord A, Harding SA. Use of the Sheathless Eaucath Is an Effective Strategy to Overcome Resistant Severe Radial Spasm. *J Interv Cardiol.* 2023 Feb 22;*2023*:2434516. doi: 10.1155/2023/2434516
14. Chyrchel M et al. Safety and Efficacy of Four Different Diagnostic Catheter Curves Dedicated to One-Catheter Technique of Transradial Coronaro-Angiography-Prospective, Randomized Pilot Study. TRACT 1: Trans RAdial CoronaryAngiography Trial 1. *J Clin Med.* 2021;*10*:4722. doi: 10.3390/jcm1020 4722
15. Burzotta F, Trani C, Hamon M, Amoroso G, Kiemeneij F. Transradial Approach for Coronary Angiography and Interventions in Patients With Coronary Bypass Grafts: Tips and Tricks. *Catheter Cardiovasc Interv.* 2008;*72*(2):263–72.
16. Tsai SC, Chen MY, Chuo SK, Wang JH. The Feasibility of Kimny Guiding Catheter for ST-Segment Elevation Myocardial Infarction. *Tzu Chi Med J.* 2021 Aug 23;*34*(1):102–6.

17. Chow J, Tan CH, Tin AS, Ong SH, Tan VH, Goh YS, Gan HW, Tan KS, Lingamanaicker J. Feasibility of Transradial Coronary Angiography and Intervention Using a Single Ikari Left Guiding Catheter for ST Elevation Myocardial Infarction. *J Interv Cardiol*. 2012 Jun;*25*(3):235–44.
18. Youssef AA, Hsieh YK, Cheng CI, Wu CJ. A Single Trans-Radial Guiding Catheter for Right and Left Coronary Angiography and Intervention. *EuroIntervention*. 2008 Jan;*3*(4):475–81. doi: 10.4244/eijv3i4a85
19. Bernat I, Aminian A, Pancholy S et al. Best Practices for the Prevention of Radial Artery Occlusion After Transradial Diagnostic Angiography and Intervention: An International Consensus Paper. *J Am Coll Cardiol Intv*. 2019;*12*:2235–46.
20. Saito S, Ikei H, Hosokawa G, Tanaka S. Influence of the Ratio Between Radial Artery Inner Diameter and Sheath Outer Diameter on Radial Artery Flow After Trans-Radial Coronary Intervention. *Catheter Cardiovasc Interv*. 1999;*46*:173–8.

Haemostasis

6

Claudio Proscia and Rodney H. Stables

6.1 INTRODUCTION

Securing safe and effective haemostasis following percutaneous transradial procedures is crucial to ensure procedural success and to reduce the rate of access-site complications. Ultimately, optimal post-procedural access-site management will positively impact nursing care requirements, length of hospital stay, patient experience, and overall care-related costs. Over the last 15 years, a variety of radial compression devices, haemostatic dressings, and techniques have been trialled. However, there is no clear consensus on the optimal radial haemostatic strategy, and wide variability is observed in clinical practice amongst centres and often within the same interventional department. This chapter discusses the technology currently available to achieve radial haemostasis, with a specific focus on haemostatic dressings. The most common post-procedural complications related to haemostasis, including bleeding, haematomas, and radial artery occlusion, are also reviewed. The chapter provides important information on patent haemostasis and its clinical implications, expedited haemostatic protocols, and adequate anticoagulation levels, in light of the most recent evidence. Finally, we propose a simplified radial haemostasis protocol to standardise practice across centres, comply with the best evidence and improve clinical outcomes for patients undergoing transradial percutaneous procedures.

DOI: 10.1201/9781003153627-6

6.2 HAEMOSTATIC METHODS

With the increasing use of the transradial route, there has been an increased demand for strategies and devices to secure radial haemostasis swiftly, safely, and cost-effectively. Dedicated air-bladder and screw-in mechanical compression devices have taken over from traditional manual compression techniques using gauze bullets, elastic bandages, and rigid wrist bands (such as the Haemoband and the RadiStop). These newer radial devices have been assessed in large-randomised trials [1–3] and are utilised routinely in clinical practice. Amongst the most commonly used are the TR band (Terumo), Helix (Vascular Perspective), TRAcelet (Medtronic), ROC-band (Cormed), Zephyr (Cordis), Safeguard and Prelude Sync (Merit Medical). They allow for direct visualisation of the radial puncture site on the wrist to detect any overt bleeding or haematoma. The compressive force applied can be adjusted gradually to manage haemostasis efficiently and safely. They are comfortable for patients and promote ambulation and independence. Manufacturer recommendations and information for use (IFU) leaflets differ between devices. Despite general recommendations on transradial artery access (TRA) [4–6], there remains a lack of standardisation of the post-procedural radial access-site management in clinical practice and the absence of a clear consensus on the optimal haemostatic time and pressure-weaning protocol.

Recent randomised trials investigated the use of haemostatic dressings applied to the puncture site in combination with radial compression devices. Various pads are currently available in clinical practice that are shown to expedite haemostasis via different mechanisms (pharmacologic, chemical, desiccation, etc.). These include potassium ferrate–based dressing (StatSeal® Advanced RAD Disc; Biolife LCC, Sarasota, Florida, USA) [7–10], kaolin-impregnated gauze (QuikClot®; Z-Medica, Wallingford, Connecticut, USA) [11], chitosan-based pad [12, 13], and thrombin-based haemostat (D-Stat; Vascular Solutions [Teleflex], Minneapolis, Minnesota, USA). The haemostatic pad with the largest amount of clinical data from randomised trials is the StatSeal (Figure 6.1). This comprises two key elements which do not enter the systemic circulation: a hydrophilic polymer and potassium ferrate (an inorganic salt). The technology is reported to dehydrate the blood at the wound site by absorbing exudate, agglomerating the blood particles, and creating a seal that stops the bleeding at the puncture site. Beneath the seal, the pH is neutral, and the blood solids and proteins continue to stack down to the arteriotomy site. Above the seal, the hydrophilic polymer exchanges protons for cations, resulting in desiccation [14]. A series of *in vitro* studies assessed the physics of compression governing the performance of the TR band alone and in conjunction with StatSeal.

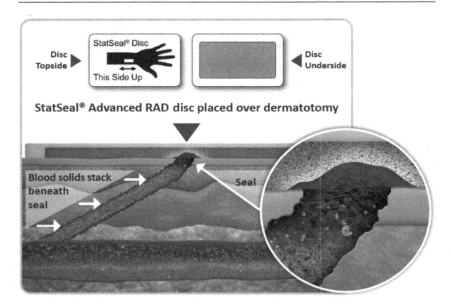

FIGURE 6.1 StatSeal Advanced RAD Disc facilitates the formation of an occlusive seal, which adheres to the wound and promotes stasis at the arteriotomy.

Reprinted with permission from Biolife LCC, Sarasota, FL, USA (http://www.statseal.com/interventional-cardiology/)

These studies suggested that the StatSeal pad might also have a mechanical role in expediting haemostasis and maintaining arterial patency by reducing intrinsic fluctuations of the TR band compression force at the access site [15]. Randomised clinical trials [7–10] demonstrate how the adjunction of the potassium-ferrate haemostatic patch to the TR band offers substantial benefits, securing haemostasis in a highly predictable and reproducible fashion, with just one hour of radial artery compression (regardless of the level of anticoagulation), across a large spectrum of patients undergoing percutaneous cardiovascular procedures. This results in quicker discharge times for planned day-care procedures and reduced likelihood of unplanned overnight stays due to prolongation of the radial care [10]. Ultimately, this translates into shorter hospital stays for patients, increased availability of bed spaces for other aspects of the service, reduced nursing requirements for radial care, and overall reduced costs of health care. Compared to the standard haemostasis with compression devices, the expedited strategy using StatSeal did not increase the low rates of access-site complications, such as clinically relevant haematomas, vascular injury requiring percutaneous/surgical intervention, and radial artery occlusion.

6.3 COMPLICATIONS OF HAEMOSTASIS

Amongst the most frequent complications associated with TRA, bleeding/ haematoma, radial artery occlusion (RAO), and arterial spasm are the most frequently observed. Occasionally, vessel perforation, dissection, pseudoaneurysm, subcutaneous granulomatous reaction, and, rarely, hand ischaemia and compartment syndrome can be observed. Previous single-centre experiences report a variable rate of haematoma between < 1% and 17%, depending on the level of anticoagulation, the modality of haemostasis used, and the size of the haematoma [3, 7–10, 16, 17]. The EArly Discharge after Transradial Stenting of CoronarY Arteries (EASY) grading system allows for a standardised and practical classification of TRA-related haematomas [16]: type I, ≤5 cm diameter; type II, ≤10 cm diameter; type III, >10 cm and below the elbow; type IV, extending above the elbow; and type V, anywhere with ischaemic threat of the hand. In most recent studies, haematomas ≥ type II average at around 2%–4%. It has been observed that while smaller haematomas (<10 cm) are usually directly related to the failure of haemostasis at the puncture site, higher-grade haematomas more often result from damage to the vessel caused by wire and/ or catheter manipulation. These are discussed further in Chapter 12.

The reported incidence of RAO ranges historically between <1% and 33%, with more recent rates observed around 2%–10% [18]. Acute postprocedural RAO rates tend to decline over the following 3 months – up to 40% reduction at 28 days [19], possibly due to spontaneous artery recanalisation. RAO is often overlooked because it runs clinically silent in most cases due to the ulnar contribution to the hand blood supply through the palmar arch. However, the chronic occlusion of the radial artery has relevant clinical consequences, with the inability to use the vessel as an access site for subsequent cardiac catheterisation or as an arterial conduit for bypass surgery or renal dialysis. Also, instrumenting the ipsilateral ulnar artery, in the case of RAO, may increase the risk of hand ischaemia. The suggested pathophysiology of RAO is linked to the mechanical injury of the vessel during arterial instrumentation, leading to endothelial damage and dysfunction, and creating a nidus for arterial thrombosis by exposing the thrombogenic connective tissue to the systemic circulation [18]. Arterial thrombosis is also favoured by blood stasis while achieving haemostasis. Various patient and procedural characteristics have been suggested to be positive predictors of RAO in different studies, such as female gender, age, smoking, diabetes mellitus, elevated serum creatinine, peripheral vascular disease, sheath-to-artery ratio > 1, absence of radial vasodilator drugs after sheath insertion (e.g., nitrates and calcium channel blockers); however, there was no consistent direction of effect of these factors on

RAO in a comprehensive review and meta-analysis of randomised trials [18]. The only independent, powerful predictors of radial patency after TRA have been identified in shorter compression times during radial haemostasis [20], routine patent haemostasis [2], and higher doses of intraprocedural heparin [18, 21]. Planned radial compression times of at least 60 minutes after a diagnostic procedure and 120–180 minutes after percutaneous coronary intervention (PCI) are currently the norm in many cardiac centres. These times are often longer due to staff clinical constraints or access-site bleeding complications. In the ARCH [10] and STAT2 [9] trials, a one-hour radial compression strategy with TR band and StatSeal secured haemostasis consistently and predictably in patients undergoing both diagnostic and angioplasty procedures, with RAO rates < 1% and no increase in the rate of vascular complications – compared to traditionally longer compression times. The level of anticoagulation and antithrombotic regimen differed largely between the two studies, but patent haemostasis was invariably used as a default strategy.

6.4 OPTIMAL ANTICOAGULANT THERAPY

With regard to anticoagulation for transradial procedures, the most recent consensus [5, 6] recommends a minimum of 5,000 U or 50 U/kg intravenous or intra-arterial unfractionated heparin (or comparable doses of enoxaparin or bivalirudin) after radial introducer sheath insertion for patients undergoing coronary angiography. This evidence was partly derived from trials with suboptimal adherence to best practices, in which patent haemostasis techniques and dedicated compression devices were not routinely used. More recently, lower doses (<5,000 IU) [9] or provisional use of heparin (i.e., no heparin administered unless unable to achieve patency during radial haemostasis) [22] were associated with a low incidence of RAO after TRA angiography (1%–5%) when patent haemostasis was maintained.

6.5 PATENT HAEMOSTASIS

Patent haemostasis is achieved by applying the maximum pressure at the radial access site to prevent bleeding while allowing antegrade flow in the artery. This should be attempted using arterial plethysmography within a few minutes of sheath removal (see Figure 6.2 for the procedural steps). For many

1. Following application of occlusive pressure via dedicated radial device and sheath removal, apply pulsoxymeter probe to the ipsilateral thumb or index

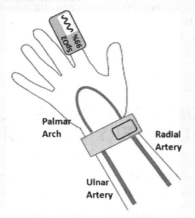

2. Observe pulsatile waveform: [∿∿∿]
3. Manually compress ulnar artery in the forearm
4. Observe flat waveform: [————]
5. Maintain firm manual ulnar pressure
6. Slowly reduce radial compression – e.g., for TR Band, deflate device (approx. 1 ml every 5 seconds)
7. Observe return of pulsatile waveform:

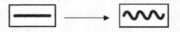

   a. Waveform observed without bleeding → **PH achieved**
   b. If any bleeding before observing waveform, increase compression slowly until bleeding stops → **PH attempted, but not achieved**

FIGURE 6.2 Patent radial haemostasis (PH) using plethysmography – procedure.

years, a different technique has been used in many centres to achieve patent haemostasis: after the application of occlusive pressure with the radial device, compression is gently released until ooze/pulsatile bleeding is seen; hence, the compression applied is minimally increased to prevent further bleeding (e.g., by inflating TR Band with 2 ml of air). This modality does not assess for antegrade flow in the artery, and it generates the minimum compression force sufficient to stop the bleeding at that stage. This may result in bleeding complications later in the haemostatic process, which could lead to unplanned prolongation of the radial care.

6.6 DETECTION OF POST-PROCEDURAL RADIAL ARTERY OCCLUSION

Previous data suggest that more than 50% of operators ignore the rate of post-procedural radial patency in their centres before discharge [18], with no form of patency check being performed. Palpation of the radial artery after successful haemostasis is, unfortunately, the most commonly used modality to assess arterial patency [23]. However, feeling a palpable radial pulse is not synonymous with patency: nearly half of the patients with acute post-procedural RAO will have a palpable radial artery [24], likely due to retrograde collateral circulation. Duplex Doppler ultrasound is currently considered the gold standard for detecting RAO. Two-dimensional ultrasound imaging allows assessment of the arterial lumen and architecture (presence of thrombus, pseudoaneurysm, dissection, etc.), and colour-doppler imaging detects the presence and direction of flow during and after ulnar artery compression. This method is not routinely used in everyday clinical practice due to limited availability, need for technical expertise, and costs.

Radial artery patency can be evaluated more timely and cost-effectively by using digital plethysmography and a modified version of the reverse Barbeau test. This technique performs comparably to duplex Doppler to assess the presence of RAO after TRA [24]. After placement of a digital sensor on the thumb (or the index finger), both radial and ulnar arteries are compressed manually (of note, in the traditional reverse Barbeau test, only the ulnar artery is compressed); loss of plethysmographic signal is recorded on the pulse-oximeter; the radial artery is then released; the return of the plethysmographic signal within 5 seconds, while manually occluding the ulnar artery, is considered evidence of radial artery patency. The *modified* version of the reverse Barbeau test reduces the likelihood of missing acutely occluded radial arteries (false negative results) compared to the traditional test. It reduces the chance that a potential third forearm artery, such as a large interosseous artery connected to the palmar arch, could generate a plethysmographic waveform despite RAO.

6.7 MANAGEMENT OF POST-PROCEDURAL RADIAL ARTERY OCCLUSION

An adjunctive non-pharmacological intervention has been shown to reduce the rate of RAO when compared to the standard PH strategy alone: ipsilateral ulnar artery compression significantly reduces the incidence of RAO, as low as 1%, with no increase in complication rates, such as haematomas or hand ischaemia. This technique can be performed by default, during radial PH, or with a provisional approach – i.e., 1-h ulnar compression, in the case of RAO detected at the end of the radial compression time. The efficacy of this strategy is thought to be related to the hemodynamic interdependence between radial and ulnar arteries via the collateralisation of the forearm and palmar circulation: the temporary occlusion of the ulnar artery creates a hyperdynamic state in the radial artery which, in turn, may improve flow-mediated dilatation, fibrinolysis, and recanalisation in the case of RAO [19, 25, 26].

If RAO is detected after radial haemostasis has been achieved, administration of subcutaneous systemic anticoagulation for one month, such as low-molecular-weight heparin or fondaparinux (prophylactic dose in case of concomitant dual antiplatelet therapy or treatment dose in the case of single antiplatelet), has also been shown to promote recanalisation [27].

6.8 OPTIMISED RADIAL HAEMOSTASIS PROTOCOL

We propose an optimised protocol for radial haemostasis as a general guideline that can be integrated into existing policies. We aim to standardise the post-procedural radial management across different centres. The safety and efficacy of this protocol, as well as its ability to reduce nursing care requirements for post-procedural radial management, have been tested in the largest single-centre randomised controlled trial comparing haemostatic dressings in transradial procedures [10]. The steps are as follows:

1. After removing the drapes from the hand and arm, clean and dry the skin around the wound thoroughly.
2. Withdraw the sheath by about one-fourth of the length.
3. Apply a small absorbent dressing with its centre lying over the point of the arterial puncture (usually 1–2 mm proximal to the skin incision) – alternatively, a haemostatic dressing, such as StatSeal, can be applied as per product IFU.
4. Place an additional bio-occlusive see-through dressing (e.g., Tegaderm) over the initial dressing to create a secure barrier to environmental contamination – and to maintain any haemostatic dressing in place.
5. Place the compression device at the arteriotomy site and secure it following the device IFU.
6. Tighten the compression device to generate occlusive pressure at the arteriotomy site while removing the radial sheath slowly and gently. In the case of a haemostatic pad, any squirt of blood from the wound or the sheath that should wet the lower surface of the dressing during sheath removal is believed to activate the pro-coagulative and haemostatic properties of the pad (Figure 6.3).
7. Perform PH with plethysmography, as described in this chapter (Figure 6.2) – if PH is not achieved successfully at this stage due to ongoing bleeding or haematoma, consider
   a. repeating #7 after 15 minutes,
   b. applying the minimum amount of pressure that prevents bleeding, or
   c. performing prophylactic concomitant ulnar compression along with #7b.
8. Observe the radial site for
   a. two hours in patients with standard absorbent dressing who received PCI (or high dose of procedural anticoagulation) and
   b. one hour in patients with haemostatic dressing (regardless of anticoagulation levels) or in patients with standard dressing and low dose of procedural anticoagulation.
   There is no routine need to adjust the compression device pressure (potentially disturbing the thrombogenic process) before first attempting full pressure release.
9. At the planned time, release *all* pressure from the device in one stage, gradually, over five to ten minutes, while closely monitoring the radial site – this facilitates prompt clinical action in case of bleeding, unlike a multi-step pressure release strategy.

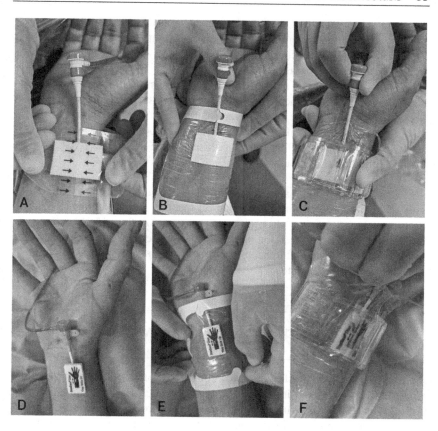

FIGURE 6.3 Proposed protocol for optimal radial haemostasis: Application of dressings and compression device. A-C: Application of standard dressing, Tegaderm and TR Band; D-F: Application of StatSeal, Tegaderm and TR Band.

 a. in case of failure of haemostasis (i.e., new bleeding or expanding haematoma), increase the radial compression to its original level, perform PH, and reattempt pressure release after one hour

 b. in case of further rebleed after 1 hour, repeat #9a every 30 minutes until successful haemostasis is achieved.

10. Once haemostasis is achieved, leave the compression device in situ for at least 15 minutes with no pressure applied to allow for quick response in case of bleeding.

11. Perform a patency check using plethysmography and the modified reverse Barbeau test, and document the outcome.

a. If there is evidence of acute RAO, consider one hour of ipsilateral ulnar artery occlusion, or one month of systemic anticoagulation, or conservative management – arrange follow-up as deemed necessary.

12. Instruct the patient to keep dressings on for a minimum of 24 hours – any attempt at replacing dressings once haemostasis has been achieved may result in new bleeding and can compromise sterility. Do not change a dressing if there is an element of blood staining. Advise the patient to avoid lifting, pushing, or extensive use of the wrist for a minimum of 24 hours.

NB: Any new/expanding haematoma should be measured, reported, and treated with adequate compression. Depending on the size and the clinical scenario, the management may vary from manual compression for ~15–20 minutes to an additional large compression device or elastic pressure bandage for longer periods. Advise the patient to keep the arm elevated and immobile. Escalate to medical staff as appropriate.

6.9 CONCLUSIONS

Safe and effective haemostasis is a key component of an optimised transradial procedure. Studies have informed the best approach to anticoagulation and haemostatic technique. With the right dose of peri-procedural heparin, modern compression/haemostatic devices, and a patent haemostatic technique, complications are minimised and efficacy is maximised. Evaluation of radial patency at the end of compression is important to detect early RAO, as it should lead to intervention in the form of ulnar compression or additional antithrombotic therapy.

REFERENCES

1. Cubero JM, Lombardo J, Pedrosa C, Diaz-Bejarano D, Sanchez B, Fernandez V, et al. Radial compression guided by mean artery pressure versus standard compression with a pneumatic device (RACOMAP). *Catheter Cardiovasc Interv.* 2009;*19229978*; 467–472.
2. Pancholy S, Coppola J, Patel T, Roke-Thomas M. Prevention of radial artery occlusion-patent hemostasis evaluation trial (PROPHET study): a randomized

comparison of traditional versus patency documented hemostasis after transradial catheterization. *Catheter Cardiovasc Interv.* 2008;*18726956*; 335–340.

3. Lavi S, Cheema A, Yadegari A, Israeli Z, Levi Y, Wall S, et al. Randomized Trial of Compression Duration After Transradial Cardiac Catheterization and Intervention. *J Am Heart Assoc.* 2017;6(2); e005029.

4. Hamon M, Pristipino C, Di Mario C, et al. Consensus document on the radial approach in percutaneous cardiovascular interventions: position paper by the European Association of Percutaneous Cardiovascular Interventions (EAPCI). *EuroIntervention.* 2013;*23354100*; 1242–1251.

5. Mason P, Shah C, Tamis-Holland V, et al. An update on radial artery access and best practices for transradial coronary angiography and intervention in acute coronary syndrome: a scientific statement from the American Heart Association. *Circ Cardiovasc Interv.* 2018;*30354598*; e000035.

6. Shroff A, Gulati R, Drachman D, et al. SCAI expert consensus statement update on best practices for transradial angiography and intervention. *Catheter Cardiovasc Interv.* 2020;*31880380*; 245–252.

7. Ayyaz U, Nazir SA, Rashid M, Kwok CS, Mubashiruddin S, Alisiddiq Z, et al. Accelerated patent hemostasis using a procoagulant disk; a protocol designed to minimize the risk of radial artery occlusion following cardiac catheterization. *Cardiovasc Revasc Med.* 2019;*29891428*; 137–142

8. Seto AH, Rollefson W, Patel MP, Suh WM, Tehrani DM, Nguyen JA, et al. Radial haemostasis is facilitated with a potassium ferrate haemostatic patch: the Statseal with TR Band assessment trial (STAT). *EuroIntervention.* 2018;*29769165*; e1236–e42.

9. Safirstein J, Tehrani D, Schussler J, Reid N, Mukerjee K, Weber L, et al. Radial hemostasis is facilitated with a potassium ferrate hemostatic patch the STAT2 trial. *JACC Cardiovasc Interv.* 2022;*35450681*; 810–819.

10. Proscia C, Kemp I, Barton J, Brown R, Stables RH. A Randomised Control Trial to Compare Conventional and Haemostatic Dressings in Radial Arterial Access: *Assessment of radial artery complications whilst achieving rapid haemostasis -ARCH trial. Int J Cardiol*, 2024, ahead of pub.

11. Roberts JS, Pastor-Cervantes JA. Comparison of hemostasis times with a kaolin-based hemostatic pad (QuikClot Radial) vs mechanical compression (TR Band) following transradial access: a pilot prospective study. *J Invasive Cardiol.* 2017; *28809724*; 328–334.

12. Roberts JS, Pastor-Cervantes JA. Comparison of hemostasis times with a chitosan-based hemostatic pad (Clo-SurPlus Radial™) vs mechanical compression (TR Band®) following transradial access: a pilot study. *Cardiovasc Revasc Med.* 2019;*30553816*; 871–874.

13. Pathan AZ, Sheikh S, Sattar S. Randomized trial comparing radial hemostasis techniques; catechol conjugated chitosan pad (InnoSEAL) versus pneumatic compression band. *Catheter Cardiovasc Interv.* 2021;*33655650*; e181–187.

14. Biolife LLC. 510(k) K080210.Section 18.3.

15. Proscia C, Keene K, Fordham T, Stables RH. An exploration of the physics of TR Band® radial compression revealing new information, critical for optimum clinical performance. *TCT Conference, Orlando FL.* 2021.

16. Bertrand OF, De Larochelliere R, Rodes-Cabau J, Proulx G, Gleeton O, Nguyen CM, et al. A randomized study comparing same-day home discharge and

abciximab bolus only to overnight hospitalization and abciximab bolus and infusion after transradial coronary stent implantation. *Circulation.* 2006;*17145988*; 2636–2643.

17. Bertrand OF, Larose E, Rodes-Cabau J, Gleeton O, Taillon I, Roy L, et al. Incidence, predictors, and clinical impact of bleeding after transradial coronary stenting and maximal antiplatelet therapy. *Am Heart J.* 2009;*19081414*, 164–169.

18. Rashid M, Kwok C, Pancholy S, Chugh S, Sasko A, Bernat I, et al. Radial artery occlusion after transradial interventions: a systematic review and meta-analysis. *J Am Heart Assoc.* 2016;*26811162*; e002686.

19. Pancholy S, Bernat I, Bertrand O, Patel T. Prevention of radialartery occlusion after transradial catheterization: the PROPHET-IIrandomized trial. *JACC Cardiovasc Interv.* 2016;*27712733*, 1992–1999.

20. Dangoisse V, Guédès A, Chenu P, et al. Usefulness of a gentle and short hemostasis using the Transradial band device after Transradial access for percutaneous coronary angiography and interventions to reduce the radial artery occlusion rate (from the prospective and randomized CRASOC I, II, and III studies). *Am J Cardiol.* 2017;*28577752*; 374–379.

21. Hahalis G, Leopoulou M, Tsigkas G, et al. Multicenter randomized evaluation of high versus standard heparin dose on incident radial arterial occlusion after transradial coronary angiography: the SPIRIT OF ARTEMIS study. *J Am Coll Cardiol Intv.* 2018;*30391389*; 2241–2250.

22. Pancholy S, Patel T. Comparison of a priori versus provisional heparin therapy on radial artery occlusion after transradial coronary angiography and patent hemostasis (from the PHARAOH study). *Am J Cardiol.* 2012;*22497680*; 173–176.

23. Shroff AR, Vidovich MI, Rao SV, Cowley M, Bertrand, OF, et al. Contemporary transradial access practices: results of the second international survey. *Catheter Cardiovasc Interv.* 2019;*30456913*; 1276–1287.

24. Pancholy S, Patel V. Comparison of diagnostic accuracy of digital plethysmography versus duplex ultrasound in detecting radial artery occlusion after transradial access. *Cardiovasc Revasc Med.* 2021;*32855082*; 52–56.

25. Bernat I, Bertrand O, Rokyta R, et al. Efficacy and safety of transient ulnar artery compression to recanalize acute radial artery occlusion after transradial catheterization. *Am J Cardiol.* 2011;*21439528*; 1698–1701.

26. Eid-Lidt G, Farjat-Pasos JI, et al. Prevention of radial artery occlusion of hemostatic methods in transradial intervention for coronary angiography. *J Am Coll Cardiol Intv.* 2022;*35589232*; 1022–1029.

27. Zankl AR, Volz C, Ivandic B, Krumsdorf U, Katus HA, Blessing E. Radial artery thrombosis following transradial coronary angiography: incidence and rationale for treatment of symptomatic patients with low-molecular-weight heparins. *Clin Res Cardiol.* 2010;*20625752*; 841–847.

Challenging Radial Cases

7

Sudhir Rathore and Fraser Witherow

7.1 RADIAL ACCESS IN COMPLEX CASES

Complex percutaneous coronary intervention (PCI) includes chronic total occlusion (CTO), left main disease, bifurcation disease, severely calcified disease, and ST elevation myocardial infarction (STEMI). All these cases can be treated via radial access [1]. PCI for complex cases often requires more guide catheter support to allow passage of wires and equipment through occlusive, severely narrowed, and calcified lesions. Additionally, complex PCI often requires a large guiding catheter to provide sufficient space to accommodate multiple wires, balloons, and other equipment simultaneously (Figure 7.1). The most important reason to choose the transfemoral artery approach (TFA) is the preferred use of large-bore (LB) guiding catheters (≥7F), which is associated with higher procedural success in CTO PCI [2]. Because of the smaller size of the radial artery, the resulting sheath-to-artery mismatch might lead to more vascular and bleeding complications [3], thereby potentially restricting the use of the radial artery for LB access.

The COLOR (Complex Large-Bore [LB] Radial) PCI [4] randomised controlled trial comparing large-bore transradial artery access (TRA) and TFA for complex coronary lesion PCI demonstrated that 7F slender TRA leads to a significant reduction in clinically relevant bleeding or vascular complications compared with 7F TFA, without any differences in crossover rates and procedural PCI success. The primary endpoint (BARC 2, 3, or 5 Bleeding or Vascular Complication Requiring Intervention of the Randomized Access Site) was observed in 19.1% of the TFA group and 3.6% in the TRA group ($p < 0.001$).

DOI: 10.1201/9781003153627-7

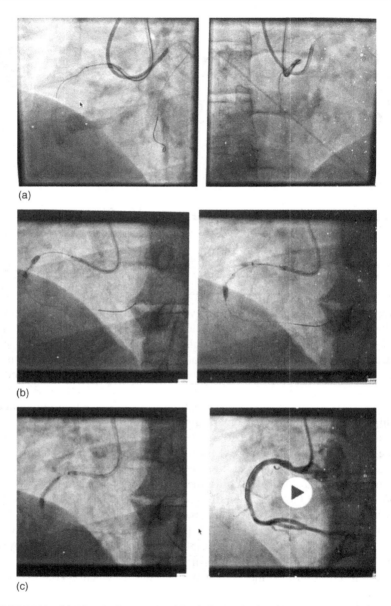

(a)

(b)

(c)

FIGURE 7.1   (a) RCA CTO PCI using biradial 7F vascular access, (b) 7F radial access treatment of severe calcific RCA stenosis with extra back up catheter and guide catheter extension support, (c) intra vascular lithotripsy and final result.

A similar benefit was achieved for procedural duration, contrast volume, and radiation exposure. CTO was the most frequently treated complex coronary lesion (58%), followed by heavy calcification (19%), left main (14%), and complex bifurcation (9%). Successful introduction of the sheath at the randomised access site occurred in 97% of the TFA group and 96% of the TRA group ($p = 0.29$). TF-to-TR crossover occurred in 2.6%, and TR-to-TF crossover occurred in 3.6% ($p = 0.56$). Dual arterial access was used in 70% of patients with CTOs.

Several other studies have examined the use of transradial access for CTO PCI. In RECHARGE (Registry of CrossBoss and Hybrid Procedures in France, the Netherlands, Belgium, and the United Kingdom), Bakker et al. [5] showed that the procedural success rate of fully transradial ($n = 306$ [24%]) and transfemoral CTO interventions ($n = 947$ [76%]) remained comparable even with increasing lesion complexity (100% vs. 99%; $p = 0.99$ [J-CTO score 0]; 97% vs. 94%; $p = 0.52$ [J-CTO score 1]; 85% vs. 88%; $p = 0.47$ [J-CTO score 2]; and 72% vs. 79%; $p = 0.17$ [J-CTO score 3]), although use of the retrograde approach was significantly lower in the transradial group (18% vs. 39%; $p < 0.01$). Rinfret et al. [3], in an early Canadian experience ($n = 42$), showed that retrograde CTO PCI is feasible with biradial access using mainly 6-F sheaths for antegrade and retrograde injections with high technical success (93%) (83% primary retrograde success) and no major in-hospital complications. In an earlier report (650 CTO PCI) from PROGRESS CTO, Alaswad et al. [6] showed similar retrograde approach use in CTO PCI with transradial approach versus transfemoral cases (50% vs. 43%; $p = 0.16$). Similarly, Rathore et al. [9] demonstrated the use of a transradial approach with success (composite of RA and RFA) compared against transfemoral cases (37% vs. 36%; $p = 0.467$). However, transradial access was more successful as a crossing technique (25% vs. 22%; $p < 0.001$), even for lesions with high complexity (46% vs. 35%; $p = 0.003$ [J-CTO score 4]; 49% vs. 40%; $p = 0.008$ [J-CTO score 5]) in comparison with transfemoral cases. Antegrade dissection re-entry techniques were less frequently used in transradial interventions (27% vs. 32%; $p = 0.002$) and were less efficient in lesions with higher complexity. The limited efficacy of antegrade dissection re-entry with transradial access may be attributed to the smaller bore access size, as in dissection re-entry techniques, more devices are likely to be used in a single catheter to facilitate wire manoeuvring and re-entry; re-entry may also require additional complex techniques, such as guide extension techniques (mother-daughter, mother-daughter-granddaughter), subintimal transcatheter withdrawal, anchoring techniques, the side-BASE technique, and so on. Kinnaird et al. [7] analysed the procedural and in-hospital outcomes of CTO PCIs using the femoral and radial approach using the British Cardiovascular Intervention Society database, demonstrating a significant decrease from 85% to 58% ($p < 0.0001$) in femoral access site use of 26,807

CTO interventions performed in the United Kingdom between 2006 and 2013. In-hospital major complications, such as death (0.2% vs. 0.1%; p = 0.027), acute myocardial infarction (MI; 0.5% vs. 0.2%; p = 0.037), and major bleeding (0.8% vs. 0.1%; $p < 0.001$), were significantly higher in trans-femoral cases, along with vascular access complications (1.5% vs. 0.5%; $p < 0.001$). Transradial CTO interventions (n = 2,748) were mostly performed with a single arterial access site (95.9%), and dual angiography was rarely performed (4.1%).

7.2 TIPS AND TRICKS FOR COMPLEX PCI CASES

The recent availability of modern slender technology, such as the thin-walled radial introducer sheath (Glidesheath Slender, Terumo, Tokyo, Japan), has the potential to overcome the anatomic limitation of TRA and to expand its use for complex PCI. It was recently shown that complex transradial (TR) PCI with a 7F Glidesheath Slender was safe and feasible, with a high rate of procedural success and a low rate of vascular complications [8]. Several observational studies have been published describing the feasibility of LB TRA for PCI of complex coronary lesions without affecting procedural success rates [2, 4, 9].

Another approach to overcome the potential challenge of using LB catheters for radial cases is the use of sheathless guiding catheters, as discussed in Section 5.5.5 (Figure 7.2). This technique has been shown to be both safe and effective in both elective and primary PCI for patients with STEMI [10]. However, the main advantage is the ability to allow transradial passage of the LB 7 or 8 Fr guide catheters that may be required for complex coronary interventions [11].

7.2.1 Sheathless Catheter-Assisted Tracking (CAT)

The radial artery is cannulated with a standard 5 or 6 Fr radial artery sheath. Diagnostic coronary angiography may be performed in the usual manner with either 5 or 6 Fr diagnostic catheters. If diagnostic images indicate that coronary intervention is required with an LB guide catheter, then the 5 or 6 Fr diagnostic catheter is removed over a J-tip (260 cm) 0.035″ guidewire positioned and secured in the ascending aorta. The introducer sheath is then also removed over

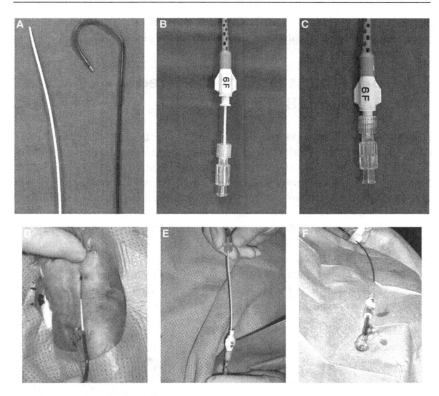

FIGURE 7.2 Dedicated sheathless guides are designed with a hydrophilic coating and dedicated introducer with a long taper (Panel A-C). This facilitates passage through the skin over a standard 0.035" wire (Panel E) and allows passage of large-bore guides (6.5F and 7.5F) even through small calibre and/or tortuous vessels. Once advanced into the ascending aorta the introducer and wire can be withdrawn and guide positioned as normal (Panel D-F).

the J-tip (260 cm) guidewire. Pressure is then applied onto the radial artery access site once the introducer sheath is removed. A 7 or 8 Fr standard guide catheter with a 5 Fr multipurpose catheter (or pigtail catheter – as these are longer than standard guiding catheters) extending beyond the tip provides a smooth transition from wire to catheter and is loaded onto the J-tip (260 cm) guidewire. This delivery system is then passed into the ascending aorta under fluoroscopic guidance. The inner 5 Fr multipurpose catheter is then removed, leaving the 7 or 8 Fr guide within the ascending aorta ready to be manoeuvred in the standard way to cannulate the coronary artery. On completion of the intervention, the guide catheter is taken out using the standard over-the-wire technique, and a haemostatic compression device is placed [12].

7.2.2 Sheathless Balloon-Assisted Tracking (BAT)

A modified version adopts the balloon-assisted technique, described previously (Section 4.7), for tortuous radial arteries where it may be difficult to pass an 0.035″ wire. A regular 0.014″ coronary interventional wire is passed under fluoroscopic guidance through a standard 5 or 6 Fr radial introducer sheath to the ascending aorta. The introducer sheath is removed, and the 7 Fr introducer without the sheath is passed over the 0.014″ wire to ensure an adequate passage has been made into the radial artery and to dilate the track (Figure 7.3). The introducer is then removed and the delivery system is then loaded onto and passed along the 0.014″ wire to the ascending aorta. The delivery system consists of an LB guide catheter with a balloon (2.5–3 mm diameter) positioned so that it protrudes partially outside the guide catheter. The balloon is then inflated to low pressure, 6–8 atmospheres. The delivery system creates a soft

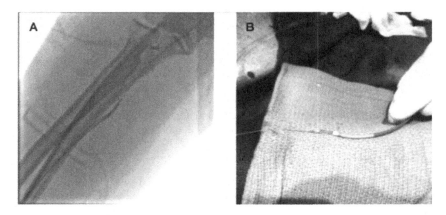

FIGURE 7.3 Balloon-assisted tracking: A: 2 mm diameter standard angioplasty balloon is loaded on a standard 0.014 wire and passed within a 6 Fr guide catheter and positioned so that half protrudes outside the guide catheter and is subsequently inflated to low pressure of 4–6 atmospheres facilitating passage of the catheter through challenging radial anatomy. B: Balloon positioned protruding from catheter and loaded onto 0.014 wire prior to introduction into radial artery.

tapered edge that passes within the radial artery. Once the delivery system has reached the ascending aorta the balloon is deflated and, along with the 0.014″ hydrophilic coronary angioplasty wire, may be changed to a standard 0.035″ guidewire providing greater support. The coronary artery is then cannulated the standard way.

7.2.3 Impact of LB Access on Hand Function

A predefined sub-study of the COLOR trial [13] assessed upper- and lower-extremity dysfunction after LB radial and femoral access. Overall, upper- and lower-extremity function did not decrease over time when LB TRA and TFA were used for complex PCI, as represented by the median Quick Disabilities of the Arm, Shoulder, and Hand score (6.8 at baseline and 2.1 at follow-up, higher is worse) and Lower-Extremity Functional Scale score (56 at baseline and 58 at follow-up, lower is worse). Clinically relevant extremity dysfunction occurred in 6% after TRA and 9% after TFA. A trend for more pronounced upper-limb dysfunction was present in female patients after LB TRA ($P = 0.05$). Lower-extremity pain at discharge was significantly higher in patients with femoral access site complications ($P = 0.02$).

Studies have shown the safety and feasibility of using LB catheters via transradial approach to successfully complete complex PCI with high success rates and lower vascular complications. Following LB TRA and TFA, self-reported upper- and lower-limb function did not deteriorate over time in most patients. Clinically relevant limb dysfunction occurs in a small minority of patients regardless of vascular access.

7.3 RADIAL ACCESS IN STEMI – TIPS AND TRICKS

Primary PCI can pose a challenge for the radial operator, as the patient may be acutely unwell or haemodynamically unstable, and expeditious vascular access is required to treat the patient as rapidly as possible. A recent meta-analysis of TRA in STEMI has shown a lower risk of all-cause mortality driven by lower bleeding complications compared with TFA [14]. TRA results in reduced vascular access and bleeding complications both as an inpatient and at 30 days following PCI.

In TRA, minimising the number of catheter changes reduces the risk of radial spasm and can speed up the procedure. To avoid multiple catheter changes, use a guide catheter that can fit both coronary ostia (such as the Ikari L3.5 or L4), which has the benefit of reducing door-to-balloon time and radiation dose, and resolves the uncertainty of which vessel is the culprit in ambiguous cases as the catheter can usually be used to visualise and then intervene on left and right coronary arteries (see Section 5.5.3) [15].

In patients with STEMI, the radial pulse can be more difficult to palpate manually as the blood pressure may be lower. If access is difficult, it is worth spending an extra minute to visualise the radial artery with ultrasound to assist with a puncture (see Section 3.6.2) rather than abandoning radial and switching to femoral access.

The incidence of patients with previous bypass grafting in STEMI is around 7%. Although STEMI due to failure of the left internal mammary artery is very rare [16], a left radial approach facilitates imaging and intervention of the native coronaries, left internal mammary, and vein grafts and should be used as the access site of choice.

There have been several studies showing that using radial access to treat STEMI patients with cardiogenic shock is superior in terms of mortality at 30 days and 1 year [17], as compared to femoral access. The radial pulse may be difficult to palpate in patients with cardiogenic shock. Despite this, it is beneficial to use the radial as it minimises bleeding risk and leaves the femoral available for a ventricular assist device or balloon pump if required. The sheath can also be used for pressure transduction post-procedure for some time while the patient is being transferred to an intensive care environment. If the radial is difficult to feel due to hypotension, a bolus of noradrenaline or metaraminol can be given to raise the blood pressure so that the artery becomes palpable. If the pressure remains low, use ultrasound to guide the puncture. If these measures fail, a femoral pulse may still be palpable, and this access site should be used to avoid delaying revascularisation.

7.4 CONCLUSIONS

Radial access is increasingly used for complex interventional cases and is associated with a reduction in complication rates. Even the most complex cases, needing enhanced support and large-diameter guide catheters, can be performed by operators familiar with the techniques needed to position LB guiding catheters.

REFERENCES

1. Sousa-Uva M, Neumann FJ, Ahlsson A, et al. 2018 ESC/EACTS Guidelines on Myocardial Revascularization. *Eur J Cardiothorac Surg.* 2019;*55*:4–90.
2. Tanaka Y, Moriyama N, Ochiai T, et al. Transradial Coronary Interventions for Complex Chronic Total Occlusions. *J Am Coll Cardiol Intv* 2017;*10*:235–43.
3. Rinfret S, Joyal D, Nguyen CM, et al. Retrograde Recanalization of Chronic Total Occlusions From the Transradial Approach; Early Canadian Experience. *Catheter Cardiovasc Interv* 2011;*78*:366–74.
4. Meijers TA, Aminian A, van Wely M, Teeuwen K, Schmitz T, Dirksen MT, Rathore S, van der Schaaf RJ, Knaapen P, Dens J, Iglesias JF, Agostoni P, Roolvink V, Hermanides RS, van Royen N, van Leeuwen MAH. Randomized Comparison Between Radial and Femoral Large-Bore Access for Complex Percutaneous Coronary Intervention. *JACC Cardiovasc Interv* 2021;*14*(12):1293–1303.
5. Bakker EJ, Maeremans J, Zivelonghi C, et al. Fully Transradial versus Transfemoral Approach for Percutaneous Intervention of Coronary Chronic Total Occlusions Applying the Hybrid Algorithm: Insights From RECHARGE Registry. *Circ Cardiovasc Interv* 2017;*10*:e005255.
6. Alaswad K, Menon RV, Christopoulos G, et al. Transradial Approach for Coronary Chronic Total Occlusion Interventions: Insights From a Contemporary Multicenter Registry. *Catheter Cardiovasc Interv* 2015;*85*:1123–9.
7. Kinnaird T, Anderson R, Ossei-Gerning N, et al. Vascular Access Site and Outcomes Among 26,807 Chronic Total Coronary Occlusion Angioplasty Cases From the British Cardiovascular Interventions Society National Database. *J Am Coll Cardiol Intv* 2017;*10*:635–44.
8. Zong B, Liu Y, Han B, Feng CG. Safety and Feasibility of a 7F Thin-Walled Sheath *via* Distal Transradial Artery Access for Complex Coronary Intervention. *Front Cardiovasc Med.* 2022 Oct 12;*9*:959197. doi: 10.3389/fcvm.2022.959197.
9. Rathore S, Hakeem A, Pauriah M, Roberts E, Beaumont A, Morris JL. A Comparison of the Transradial and the Transfemoral Approach in Chronic Total Occlusion Percutaneous Coronary Intervention. *Catheter Cardiovasc Interv* 2009;*73*:883–7.
10. Miyasaka M, Tada N, Kato S, et al. Sheathless Guide Catheter in Transradial Percutaneous Coronary Intervention for ST-Segment Elevation Myocardial Infarction. *Catheter Cardiovasc Interv.* 2016;*87*:1111–17. doi: 10.1002/ccd.26144
11. From AM, Gulati R, Prasad A et al. Sheathless Transradial Intervention Using Standard Guide Catheters. *Catheter Cardiovasc Interv.* 2010;*76*:911–16. doi: 10.1002/ccd.22742
12. Li Q, He Y, Jiang R, et al. Using Sheathless Standard Guiding Catheters for Transradial Percutaneous Coronary Intervention to Treat Bifurcation Lesions. *Exp Clin Cardiol* 2013;*18*:73–6.
13. Meijers TA, Aminian A, van Wely M, Teeuwen K, Schmitz T, Dirksen MT, Rathore S, van der Schaaf RJ, Knaapen P, Dens J, Iglesias JF, Agostoni P, Roolvink V, Hermanides RS, van Royen N, van Leeuwen MAH. Extremity Dysfunction After Large-Bore Radial and Femoral Arterial Access. *J Am Heart Assoc.* 2022;*11*:e023691. DOI: 10.1161/JAHA.121.023691

14. Sattar Y, Majmundar M, Ullah W, Mamtani S, Kumar A, Robinson S, Zghouzi M, Mir T, Dhamrah U, Al-Khadra Y, Pacha HM. Outcomes of Transradial versus Transfemoral Access of Percutaneous Coronary Intervention in STEMI: Systematic Review and Updated Meta-Analysis. *Expert Rev Cardiovasc Ther.* 2021 May 4;*19*(5):433–44.

15. Torii S, Fujii T, Murakami T, Nakazawa G, Ijichi T, Nakano M, Ohno Y, Shinozaki N, Yoshimachi F, Ikari Y. Impact of a Single Universal Guiding Catheter on Door-to-Balloon Time in Primary Transradial Coronary Intervention for ST Segment Elevation Myocardial Infarction. *Cardiovasc Interv Th.* 2017 Apr;*32*:114–19.

16. Kohl LP, Garberich RF, Yang H, Sharkey SW, Burke MN, Lips DL, Hildebrandt DA, Larson DM, Henry TD. Outcomes of Primary Percutaneous Coronary Intervention in ST-Segment Elevation Myocardial Infarction Patients With Previous Coronary Bypass Surgery. *J Am Coll Cardiol Intv.* 2014 Sep;*7*(9):981–7.

17. Ahsan MJ, Ahmad S, Latif A, Lateef N, Ahsan MZ, Abusnina W, Nathan S, Altin SE, Kolte DS, Messenger JC, Tannenbaum M. Transradial versus Transfemoral Approach for Percutaneous Coronary Intervention in Patients With ST-Elevation Myocardial Infarction Complicated by Cardiogenic Shock: A Systematic Review and Meta-Analysis. *Eur Heart J Qual Care Clin Outcomes.* 2022 Nov;*8*(6):640–50.

Transradial Access in Special Circumstances

8

Gurbir Bhatia and Helen Routledge

8.1 INTRODUCTION

This chapter provides an overview of the use of radial access for coronary procedures in specific and more challenging circumstances. We discuss the advantages, considerations, and potential limitations of the radial approach in the population of patients with renal failure and those with difficult body habitus. In these groups, we emphasise the importance of individual patient assessment and the role of experienced interventional cardiologists in decision-making. It aims to equip cardiologists with the knowledge and understanding needed to perform radial procedures safely in these high-risk patient groups without defaulting to the femoral approach. It also aims to describe the use of the upper limb when undertaking right heart catheterisation and structural heart procedures.

DOI: 10.1201/9781003153627-8

8.2 RADIAL ACCESS IN PATIENTS WITH RENAL FAILURE

It is well recognised that cardiovascular disease is the principal cause of death in patients with chronic kidney disease (CKD). CKD is associated with atherosclerotic vascular disease, and this is not merely due to background factors, such as diabetes and hypertension, that are common in both conditions. Furthermore, the risk of vascular disease and associated fatal events is increased as the severity of CKD progresses. Cardiologists will be familiar with the fact that coronary findings on angiography are likely to be more complex with higher rates of calcified lesions. Against this background, diagnosis, investigation, and treatment of coronary disease in CKD patients is nuanced due to factors such as atypical presenting symptoms, inaccurate predictive models, less accurate non-invasive testing, and uncertainties regarding optimal therapies; it should be appreciated that large trials have historically excluded CKD patients so that treatment of coronary artery disease in this sizeable population subset is not so well grounded in the evidence base that may apply to the general population [1, 2].

8.2.1 Clinical Outcomes and Evidence Base

It is well recognised that invasive coronary investigation and treatment carries a risk of renal injury, often but not exclusively related to contrast volume. In the United States, the National Cardiovascular Data Registry reported an incidence of acute kidney injury (AKI) of 7.1% among almost a million patients undergoing percutaneous coronary intervention (PCI) over a two-year period [3]. Independent predictors did include higher contrast volume, along with age and diabetes, but stronger predictors included anaemia, urgent and emergent presentation, shock, and baseline CKD. Moreover, patients with AKI, and especially those requiring dialysis, were independently associated with significantly worse in-hospital outcomes, including bleeding, myocardial infarction, and death. The study did not report on the impact of vascular access sites; at the time that these data were being collated (2009–11), the rates of transradial PCI in the United States were low. Subsequently, a registry of over 80,000 PCI procedures in Michigan was compiled between 2010–12, with transradial access accounting for just over 10%. Transradial access was associated with a significantly lower risk of bleeding, as might be expected, but also a lower risk of AKI, which did not appear to be due to the lower bleeding risk [4]. Nevertheless, a retrospective observational study of PCI patients in Japan

[5] demonstrated that patients who experienced periprocedural bleeding were more likely to develop suspected contrast-related AKI and that this was related to the severity of bleeding. Interestingly, a pre-specified analysis from a large, randomised study assessing the effect of radial access versus femoral access on AKI in over 8,000 acute PCI recipients [6] reported a significant reduction in AKI with transradial access performed by experienced operators. Patients with a higher pre-procedural risk of AKI seemed to benefit from transradial access. Although bleeding was an independent predictor of AKI, and bleeding was lower in the transradial group, major bleeding rates were low and felt unlikely to explain the AKI overall. Other putative mechanisms underlying potential radial advantages may include avoiding disruption of abdominal aortic atheromatous plaques and subsequent cholesterol embolisation to the renal arteries.

In the population with established CKD, a meta-analysis of five observational studies comprising over 7,000 patients has assessed whether transradial PCI carries advantages over femoral access in patients with CKD (eGFR < 30mL/min/1.73m^2), 90% of whom had end-stage disease [7]. The authors reported significantly lower rates of bleeding, blood transfusions, and all-cause mortality with transradial access. In addition, contrast volumes were lower, and stroke rates were not increased compared to the femoral approach.

8.2.2 Pre-procedural Considerations in Patients with Renal Failure

As with all patients, the first question should be whether the patient with established CKD needs to have invasive angiography/PCI. Specific issues clouding the picture in the CKD population relate to a smaller evidence base for treatment [1]. In the case of acute ST segment elevation myocardial infarction, it will generally be the case that primary PCI should be performed for myocardial salvage and symptom relief. In non-ST segment elevation acute coronary syndromes, it may be argued that an initial invasive approach in the face of end-stage renal failure may not be ideal and that this can be deferred and performed if there are recurrent symptoms refractory to medical therapies or haemodynamic or electrical instability. The long-term benefits of revascularisation in this group of patients are also less clear. In chronic coronary syndromes, the ISCHEMIA-CKD study has provided some insight [8]. This study demonstrated no benefit of an initial invasive approach in over 800 patients with advanced CKD and moderate or severe ischaemia (but without disabling symptoms, without recent acute presentations, and without severe left ventricular systolic dysfunction): there was no reduction in the risk of death or non-fatal myocardial infarction with PCI against medical therapy. The separate question of what exactly constitutes optimal medical therapy in CKD patients requires further clarification.

If a plan is made to perform invasive coronary procedures on the patient with CKD, then the responsible cardiologist should aim to reduce the risk of contrast-related kidney injury, regardless of the procedural access site. Assessment of risk can utilise dedicated scoring systems [9], taking into account patient-specific factors, such as eGFR and the presence of hypotension or heart failure, along with procedural factors. Ensuring patients are adequately hydrated remains important, and the use of intravenous saline administration is a simple measure that should be taken. Striving to limit volumes of contrast using ultra-low or zero-contrast strategies has garnered much attention in an age in which the use of intra-coronary physiology and imaging are commonplace [10].

While the exact mechanisms driving the renal advantages with transradial access in the general and CKD population are unclear, there does appear to be a distinct benefit. When taken together with the general advantages of quicker ambulation and shorter hospital stay, it would appear to be a strong argument favouring the radial approach. However, some cardiologists and nephrologists will balk at the idea of using transradial access due to understandable concerns that any subsequent radial artery occlusion or endothelial injury will impact negatively on the ability to construct radio-cephalic arteriovenous fistulae for haemodialysis in those with, or in those likely to progress to, end-stage renal failure. Such fistulae in the distal arm are generally felt to be the first choice when constructing vascular access [11]. It is unclear if previous radial artery cannulation without occlusion is associated with diminished long-term patency rates of radio-cephalic fistulae, and this would represent a valuable area of future research. Similarly, some CKD patients may end up requiring surgical revascularisation, and proponents of total arterial grafting may prefer to use transfemoral access for diagnostic angiography, thereby allowing the harvesting of a healthy, uninjured radial artery. The authors' practice is to aim to use transradial access wherever possible due to increased bleeding risks in renal failure patients. However, this is an important concern and should prompt a discussion between cardiologist, nephrologist, and patient.

8.2.3 Technical Considerations

When embarking upon transradial procedures in the CKD population, operators should be wary of certain anatomical difficulties which may be encountered. CKD patients are more likely to have background hypertension, which may lead to higher rates of vessel tortuosity. Similarly, demographic factors may be important: South Asian patients are more likely to have CKD by virtue of diabetic status, and such patients have smaller radial artery diameters, which could be prone to spasm, so operators should be familiar with measures to reduce this. With altered calcium metabolism in CKD, vessels may be more prone to calcification. This may hinder vessel puncture and sheath placement. The use of ultrasonography may be a useful means by which to measure radial artery dimensions and to ensure successful radial artery puncture in non-calcified portions.

Accepting that there may be a need to use radial arteries for arterio venous fistula construction makes it imperative that operators endeavour to avoid radial artery occlusion, which may be more common in the CKD population [12]. Recognised measures would include avoiding large sheaths, ensuring appropriate anticoagulation, using patent haemostasis techniques after the procedure is completed, or using distal radial access. The fact that renal failure patients are likely to have more complex, calcific coronary artery lesions may be a factor influencing operators to use larger sheaths transfemorally. In recent years, the use of slender, thin-walled radial artery sheaths has allowed for sheath insertion in those with smaller calibre vessels, and we would encourage the use of such equipment in the renal population. Experienced operators will also be able to employ assisted tracking techniques to advance larger guiding catheters up the arm, along with using guide-extension systems. These techniques mitigate difficulties in using transradial access to perform complex coronary interventions in both the general and the CKD populations.

8.2.4 Conclusion

Observational data have shown that transradial access PCI has advantages over the femoral approach in patients with CKD. This is unlikely to be explained by a reduction in bleeding alone, although this is clearly important. Performing invasive coronary procedures in this group of patients requires careful and individualised planning, taking the patient's and their nephrologist's thoughts into account. Transradial procedures should be performed by experienced operators with access to contemporary equipment and optimised techniques in order to maximise procedural success and safety, and to conserve radial artery patency for future use.

8.3 RADIAL ACCESS IN EXTREMES OF STATURE

Experienced transradial operators will readily recognise the challenges posed by patients with certain body habitus – for example, those with short stature or very elevated body mass index (BMI). Broadly speaking, all the advantages of transradial access in the general population are applicable to these groups of patients. Indeed, it is strongly argued that those with the highest BMI stand to gain the most given their inherently increased bleeding risks from transfemoral procedures [13].

It is incumbent on all operators to be familiar with the details of non-emergent patients prior to their arrival on the table. This should include knowledge of their body habitus, which may influence and complicate the planned procedure, not to mention the impact on revascularisation decisions.

It has long been recognised that patient height can impact transradial procedures. For example, shorter height has been found to be associated with tortuosity of the right subclavian artery [14, 15], thereby prolonging procedures performed with right radial access. A similar association has been noted for elevated BMI [14]. These factors may be further compounded by older age, female gender [16], and the presence of background hypertension. Thus, the experienced operator can anticipate potential difficulties due to subclavian artery tortuosity when patients enter the catheterisation laboratory.

One potentially useful way to mitigate difficulties due to such body habitus is to consider using left rather than right radial access. Historically, observational studies, albeit with methodological flaws and inconsistencies, have generally shown longer procedural times and higher radiation exposures with right radial access compared to transfemoral approaches. While some of these drawbacks can be overcome with greater experience, meta-analysis of randomised, observational studies using left radial access has been shown to reduce radiation doses compared to the right radial [17]. Some of the increase in dose may relate to the placement of the lead shielding; some may relate to more frequently coming across subclavian tortuosity with right-sided access.

A small, randomised observational study addressed whether left vs. right radial access could provide advantages in patients who may be expected to provide procedural challenges from the outset (due to short stature, female gender, higher age, and the presence of background hypertension) [18]. Interestingly, the radiation parameters measured did not differ significantly between the left and right radial approaches. Another factor to take on board is that of operator comfort. One study addressed this issue when considering left vs. right radial access [19]. Although the operators' radiation doses were reduced with left radial access, this was countered by higher levels of discomfort reported by operators, especially when performing procedures for patients with the highest BMI.

Operators should carefully review previous coronary imaging data for all patients due to enter the catheter laboratory for repeated procedures. Occasionally, we may see that selective catheter engagement has been hindered by the presence of right subclavian tortuosity. Operators may opt to default to left radial access, but often, this tortuosity can be overcome by asking patients to inspire deeply to straighten the angle between the innominate artery and ascending aorta. The authors have a low threshold to use alternative diagnostic catheters to those that were unsuccessful previously. In the case of right coronary intubation, we prefer to use catheters with a longer distal tip than the standard JR4 – e.g., Amplatz catheters (AR1 or 2, or AL1). If using left radial access, engagement of the left coronary with a JL4 catheter rather than JL 3.5 is preferable, as in most patients, the course will be like that with transfemoral access. For taller patients undergoing right radial procedures, a JL4 may also be preferable, as its tip is likely to sit more coaxially in the left main stem, whereas the JL3.5 tip may lie at the roof of the left main stem, risking dissection. When faced with severe thoracic vessel tortuosity, it is worth leaving the 0.035" guidewire in diagnostic and, indeed, guiding catheters prior to manipulation and engagement to reduce the risk of kinking. Ensuring availability of a range of potentially useful catheter shapes in a size compatible with the sheath used is a key step when embarking on such a procedure.

It may also follow that shorter patients are more likely to have smaller calibre radial arteries [20]. Consequently, accessing these vessels with larger calibre sheaths may increase the risk of spasm and subsequent radial artery occlusion. Simple strategies to reduce spasm include minimising sheath calibres, administration of sedation and intra-arterial vasodilator drugs, and even using hydrophilic catheters.

Future advances may come from the routine use of bilateral ultrasound scanning to assess radial artery dimensions to determine which side to use, along with the use of left distal transradial access (see Chapter 10), which may facilitate improvements in patient and operator comfort.

Finally, traditional teaching has promoted avoidance of performing transradial procedures in such patient groups early in one's learning curve. Accordingly, procedural success and safety in this subset of the population will likely be enhanced if performed by experienced operators rather than more junior trainees.

8.3.1 Right Heart Catheterisation

Cardiac catheterisation for hemodynamic evaluation was historically a routine reason for referral to the invasive cardiologist. Measurement of left- and right-sided heart pressures and the pressure in the pulmonary arteries was an essential diagnostic tool. At the same time, pulmonary artery catheterisation was commonplace for hemodynamic monitoring in the intensive care unit. In very many circumstances, progress over the last two decades in cardiac monitoring and non-invasive imaging, in particular echocardiography and cardiac magnetic resonance techniques, have negated the need for invasive pressure measurements. Roles for right heart catheterisation remain, however, and can broadly be categorised as follows:

- Diagnosis of pulmonary hypertension
- Diagnosis of pericardial constriction/restrictive cardiomyopathy
- Interrogation of presumed intracardiac shunt
- During or prior to structural intervention
- Pre- and post-transplant assessment
- Cardiac biopsy

8.3.2 Indications for Right Heart Catheterisation

Direct measurement of pulmonary artery pressure remains the gold standard for the diagnosis of pulmonary hypertension. In contrast to imaging techniques, and although it will still vary with loading conditions, no assumptions are made in obtaining an absolute value. By measurement of pulmonary capillary wedge pressure, additional information is gained as to the aetiology of the elevated pressure, broadly differentiating between pre-capillary hypertension and that due to left-sided heart disease. Invasive measurement in the cardiac catheter laboratory also allows for pulmonary angiography and acute vasodilator testing, although these are predominantly undertaken in specialist centres as part of a full structured protocol for the investigation of the patient with definite pulmonary arterial hypertension.

In confirmation of restriction or constriction, again now usually suggested by advanced non-invasive imaging modalities, a careful protocol involving simultaneous measurement of left- and right-chamber pressures must be adhered to, and avoidance of volume depletion pre-investigation is necessary. Oxygen saturation samples are obtained alongside pressure measurements in shunt assessment, the investigation of structural heart disease, and measurement of cardiac output. In valvular or congenital heart disease, ambiguous or discordant imaging measurements may prompt a request for right heart catheterisation, but it is no longer part of the standard workup for surgery. The presence of pulmonary hypertension adds to peri-operative risk, and the severity of mitral stenosis, particularly in the presence of other valve lesions, is perhaps the most common clarification required. Transplant workup hinges on measurement of the transpulmonary gradient and calculation and manipulation of pulmonary vascular resistance.

Finally, endomyocardial biopsy via right heart catheterisation has been used most commonly post-cardiac transplant to look for rejection. It may be indicated in diagnostic workup for infiltrative cardiomyopathy and acute heart failure due to myocarditis to determine the treatment pathway, but as the information derived from cardiac magnetic resonance imaging increases, the absolute indications for biopsy decrease.

8.3.3 Antecubital Fossa Access for Right Heart Catheterisation

Despite the first right heart catheter being undertaken infamously from the arm by Werner Forssmann using a urethral catheter to cannulate his own antecubital vein [21], the femoral vein has most often been used to access the right heart in patients in the catheterisation laboratory. This remains the case in many laboratories, even in those undergoing coronary angiography via the radial artery. In contrast, post-transplant and on the intensive care unit, the right heart is more often accessed via the internal jugular vein. By far, the safest approach is to enter the circulation via an antecubital vein. The benefits of avoiding a femoral approach in these patients require little further explanation but include earlier ambulation and avoidance of the need to lie flat, which is important to the breathless patient. The risk of inadvertent femoral arterial puncture in this population, many of whom benefit from uninterrupted anticoagulation, is negated. Difficulty and risk in femoral venous cannulation are exacerbated by volume depletion ("collapsed veins") as a result of fasting and diuretic therapy in this cohort. The advantage of access via the antecubital vein over femoral access also extends to the operator. The ease of passage of a catheter to the pulmonary artery from the right or left upper limb is remarkable to the cardiologist who has at any time struggled from the femoral route. Coronary angiography is often, though not always, a part of the full diagnostic procedure; thus, access to only a single draped and cleaned limb is required.

8.3.4 Anatomy

The superficial veins in the antecubital fossa are found in a predictable configuration in 80% of patients, with four common variations in the remainder. The usual pattern is where the medial vein of the forearm (median antebrachial vein) is connected by the terminal branches of the median cephalic and basilic vein at the elbow to continue as the cephalic and basilic vein in the upper arm. These vessels drain into the axillary then subclavian vein which gives easy access to the heart.

Access to the right heart from the superior vena cava is easiest from the basilic vein found in the medial aspect (ulnar side) of the antecubital fossa. The basilic vein usually has a direct straight path into the axillary vein. The cephalic vein enters the axillary at a more acute angle but can commonly be navigated (occasionally with the aid of a guidewire) in cases where the basilic is less well palpated. There is rarely important tortuosity en route to the superior vena cava and failure to navigate this route or to need to crossover to an alternative access is uncommon [22].

In contrast, the femoral vein lies in close proximity to the femoral nerve and artery. This anatomical relationship confers more risk of adverse events associated with catheterisation. In addition to bleeding, infection, and pseudoaneurysm, the additional risks of cannulation of ipsilateral femoral vein and artery for cardiac catheterisation include the possibility of iatrogenic arteriovenous fistula formation.

8.3.5 Technique of Right Heart Catheterisation via Antecubital Vein

Pre-procedure the patient should be well hydrated and ideally not fasted. Anxiolytic medication, such as small doses of intravenous benzodiazepine, are recommended pre-cannulation, particularly for radial artery cannulation, but deep sedation should be avoided for its effects on hemodynamics.

Positioning of the patient is similar to that for coronary angiography via the radial artery, but a moment of thought regarding placement of the, ideally, four (but possibly two) holed drape to provide two sterile fields over right or left radial and brachial areas and a working space is needed. A tourniquet can be positioned but not tightened on the upper arm before cleaning and draping. Identification of the best vein to cannulate is again easiest before cleaning and covering the arm and injecting a local anaesthetic (this can also be aided by using ultrasound). As outlined earlier, superior vena cava access, with the least tortuosity, is better from the more medial of the antecubital veins. If this is not palpable or accessible, then a lateral vein can be used, but a guidewire may be needed to navigate the angle. Following venous cannulation, the tourniquet is removed, and Seldinger access with a standard short radial sheath is the most practical approach for a study in the cardiac catheter laboratory such that a sheath with a haemostatic valve can be placed for the procedure. The sheath is flushed and secured with a dressing, while radial artery access can then be obtained.

For access to the right heart and pulmonary tree, the choice of catheter may be determined by availability, and a standard 5 French multipurpose diagnostic catheter will usually suffice. This will allow navigation to the right heart with a 0.035" guidewire if needed. Any resistance at all is abnormal and must be investigated with a venogram to determine if caused by tortuosity or venous occlusion. A planned biopsy may require a larger calibre guiding catheter. The alternative for a diagnostic procedure, allowing pressure and saturation monitoring, is a 5F Swan Ganz (balloon-tipped catheter with a flushable central lumen). The latter will usually "float" with ease from the right atrium through to either pulmonary artery with inflation of the balloon. Subsequent measurement of pulmonary capillary wedge pressure is achieved by re-inflating the balloon in a vessel small enough to occlude. The measurement of transpulmonary gradient is seamlessly achieved by recording mean pressure during balloon deflation. The disadvantage of the 5F Swan Ganz device is the smaller central lumen such that if a guidewire is needed to navigate any peripheral tortuosity, then a 0.014 coronary guidewire is needed. Frequent aspiration and flushing between measurements avoid damping or underestimation of right heart pressures.

A practised and reasonably standardised protocol should then be used after flushing and zeroing all transducers to obtain pressure measurements in the pulmonary artery (PA), pulmonary capillary wedge pressure (PCWP), simultaneous PCWP and left ventricular pressure (LV) (with a pigtail from the right radial), pullback from PCWP to PA, simultaneous PA and LV pressures (and wedge position), pullback to right ventricle (RV), simultaneous RV and LV pressure, pullback to right atrium (RA) pressure, simultaneous RA and LV pressure. Pressure measurements should be made consistently in end expiration to minimise respiratory variation and over several cycles, particularly in those patients with atrial fibrillation. The catheter can then be repositioned for saturation measurements, with flushing in between, where required. Pulmonary angiography or cardiac output measurements may then be added on before removal of the right heart catheter and proceeding to coronary angiography where appropriate. Removal of a 5 French venous sheath from the antecubital fossa can be undertaken in the recovery area, with haemostasis easily achieved with manual compression.

In cases where physiological manipulation is required, for example mitral stenosis of uncertain severity, patient exercise may be undertaken to clarify the situation. With upper-limb venous access the patient can be asked to perform straight leg raises to see if this can increase transmitral gradients.

8.3.6 Clinical Applications and Evidence

Antecubital fossa access for right heart catheterisation is by far the most practical approach when left heart catheterisation is undertaken via the radial artery and in a cardiac catheter suite set-up for ambulatory patients undergoing diagnostic procedures (the "radial lounge"). In some cases of respiratory pathology, pulmonologists will require the right heart catheter alone, and this can be done minimally invasively in the ambulatory patient. Avoiding the femoral will be most beneficial when studying the anticoagulated patient, likely those with pulmonary hypertension, mitral valve disease, atrial fibrillation associated with structural heart disease or cardiomyopathy, who can safely continue medication uninterrupted [23].

A decrease in discomfort, recovery time, and bleeding complications are clear to anyone switching to an upper-limb approach for right heart catheterisation. For the team, the learning curve in switching from a femoral approach is less marked than for coronary procedures. In the authors' experience, most operators, whether trainees or long-established cardiologists, find this approach more straightforward. A retrospective comparison of the femoral and forearm approaches for left and right heart catheters in 296 patients in Japan demonstrated a shorter procedure time from the upper limb. All procedures were successful and free of complications other than one pseudoaneurysm occurring in the femoral group [24]. In the United States, 175 femoral procedures were compared with 105 radial cases undertaken by the same four operators. Procedural durations were five minutes shorter via the upper limb, and access site complications occurred in 12 femoral but no radial patients [25]. Again retrospectively, but in keeping with the aforementioned, a change in practice was observed in one US centre from central venous access to antecubital fossa access over a four-year period with shorter procedure times and a reduction from 3% to 0% complication rate [22].

8.3.7 Conclusions and Future Direction

The need for right heart catheterisation procedures has diminished in number but remains an essential skill for cardiologists and one that must be acquired and understood by trainees. There will remain conditions and scenarios where the definitive diagnosis and management plan depend upon results obtained invasively. Access to the right heart by colleagues in advanced heart failure (for remote PA pressure monitoring), electrophysiology, and, increasingly, for structural interventions will continue, and although it is unlikely that upper-limb access will become appropriate for all these, there are likely modifications to the procedures which may involve the upper-limb approach. Reduction in the risk of right heart catheter procedures and the relative speed and ease of passage of catheters into the pulmonary circulation from the upper limb are important benefits of the antecubital fossa approach compared to historic use of the femoral or internal jugular veins.

REFERENCES

1. Sarnak M, Amann K, Bangalore S, et al. Chronic Kidney Disease and Coronary Artery Disease. *J Am Coll Cardiol.* 2019 Oct;*74*(14):1823–38. doi: 10.1016/j.jacc.2019.08.1017

2. Schuett K, Marx N, Lehrke M. The Cardio-Kidney Patient: Epidemiology, Clinical Characteristics and Therapy. *Circ Res.* 2023 Apr 14;*132*(8):902–14. doi: 10.1161/CIRCRESAHA.122.321748

3. Tsai T, Patel U, Chang T, et al. Contemporary Incidence, Predictors, and Outcomes of Acute Kidney Injury in Patients Undergoing Percutaneous Coronary Interventions. *J Am Coll Cardiol Intv.* 2014 Jan;*7*(1):1–9. doi: 10.1016/j.jcin.2013.06.016

4. Kooiman J, Seth M, Dixon S, et al. Risk of Acute Kidney Injury After Percutaneous Coronary Interventions Using Radial versus Femoral Vascular Access: Insights From the Blue Cross Blue Shield of Michigan Cardiovascular Consortium. *Circ Cardiovasc Interv.* 2014 Apr;*7*(2):190–8. doi: 10.1161/CIRCINTERVENTIONS.113.000778

5. Ohno Y, Maekawa Y, Miyata H, et al. Impact of Periprocedural Bleeding on Incidence of Contrast-Induced Acute Kidney Injury in Patients Treated With Percutaneous Coronary Intervention. *J Am Coll Cardiol.* 2013 Oct;*62*(14):1260–6. doi: 10.1016/j.jacc.2013.03.086

6. Andò G, Cortese B, Russo F, et al. Acute Kidney Injury After Radial or Femoral Access for Invasive Acute Coronary Syndrome Management. *J Am Coll Cardiol.* 2017 May; *69*(21):2592–603. doi: 10.1016/j.jacc.2017.02.070

7. Latif A, Ahsan MJ, Mirza MM, et al. Meta-Analysis of Transradial Versus Transfemoral Access for Percutaneous Coronary Intervention in Patients With Chronic Kidney Disease. *Am J Cardiol.* 2021 Oct 15;*157*:8–14. doi: 10.1016/j.amjcard.2021.07.018

8. Bangalore S, Maron DJ, O'Brien SM, et al. ISCHEMIA-CKD Research Group. Management of Coronary Disease in Patients with Advanced Kidney Disease. *N Engl J Med.* 2020 Apr 23;*382*(17):1608–18. doi: 10.1056/NEJMoa1915925

9. Mehran R, Owen R, Chiarito M, et al. A Contemporary Simple Risk Score for Prediction of Contrast-Associated Acute Kidney Injury After Percutaneous Coronary Intervention: Derivation and Validation From an Observational Registry. *Lancet.* 2021 Nov 27;*398*(10315):1974–83. doi: 10.1016/S0140-6736(21)02326-6

10. Ali ZA, Escaned J, Dudek D, et al. Strategies for Renal Protection in Cardiovascular Interventions. *Korean Circ J.* 2022 Jul;*52*(7):485–95. doi: 10.4070/kcj.2022.0093

11. Alnahhal KI, Rowse J, Kirksey L. The Challenging Surgical Vascular Access Creation. *Cardiovasc Diagn Ther.* 2023 Feb 28;*13*(1):162–72. doi: 10.21037/cdt-22-560

12. Tsigkas G, Papanikolaou A, Apostolos A, et al. Preventing and Managing Radial Artery Occlusion following Transradial Procedures: Strategies and Considerations. *J Cardiovasc Dev Dis.* 2023 Jun 30;*10*(7):283. doi: 10.3390/jcdd10070283

13. Hibbert B, Simard T, Wilson KR, et al. Transradial versus Transfemoral Artery Approach for Coronary Angiography and Percutaneous Coronary Intervention in the Extremely Obese. *JACC Cardiovasc Interv.* 2012 Aug;*5*(8):819–26. doi: 10.1016/j.jcin.2012.04.009

14. Cha KS, Kim MH, Kim HJ. Prevalence and Clinical Predictors of Severe Tortuosity of Right Subclavian Artery in Patients Undergoing Transradial Coronary Angiography. *Am J Cardiol.* 2003 Nov 15;*92*(10):1220–2. doi: 10.1016/j.amjcard.2003.07.038

15. Roeschl T, Jano AM, Fochler F, et al. Prevalence and Predictors of Difficult Vascular Anatomy in Forearm Artery Access for Coronary Angiography and PCI. *Sci Rep.* 2022 Jul 29;*12*(1):13060. doi: 10.1038/s41598-022-17435-1

16. Tröbs M, Achenbach S, Plank PM, et al. Predictors of Technical Failure in Transradial Coronary Angiography and Intervention. *Am J Cardiol.* 2017 Nov 1;*120*(9):1508–13. doi: 10.1016/j.amjcard.2017.07.049

17. Xia SL, Zhang XB, Zhou JS, Gao X. Comparative Efficacy and Safety of the Left versus Right Radial Approach for Percutaneous Coronary Procedures: A Meta-Analysis Including 6870 Patients. *Braz J Med Biol Res.* 2015 Aug;*48*(8):743–50. doi: 10.1590/1414-431X20154571

18. Shah B, Burdowski J, Guo Y, et al. Effect of Left versus Right Radial Artery Approach for Coronary Angiography on Radiation Parameters in Patients With Predictors of Transradial Access Failure. *Am J Cardiol.* 2016 Aug 15;*118*(4):477–81. doi: 10.1016/j.amjcard.2016.05.039

19. Kado H, Patel A, Suryadevara S, et al. Operator Radiation Exposure and Physical Discomfort During a Right versus Left Radial Approach for Coronary Interventions. *J Am Coll Cardiol Intv.* 2014 Jul;*7*(7):810–16. doi: 10.1016/j.jcin.2013.11.026

20. Giannopoulos G, Raisakis K, Synetos A, et al. A Predictive Score of Radial Artery Spasm in Patients Undergoing Transradial Percutaneous Coronary Intervention. *Int J Cardiol.* 2015 Jun 1;*188*:76–80. doi: 10.1016/j.ijcard.2015.04.024

21. Forssmann W. Die Sondierung des rechten Herzens. *Klinische Wochenschrift.* 1929;*8*:2085–7.

22. Shah S, Boyd G, Pyne CT, et al. Right Heart Catheterization Using Antecubital Venous Access: Feasibility, Safety and Adoption Rate in a Tertiary Center. *Catheter Cardiovasc Interv.* 2014 Jul 1;*84*(1):70–4. doi: 10.1002/ccd.25249

23. Lo TS, Buch AN, Hall IR, et al. Percutaneous Left and Right Heart Catheterization in Fully Anticoagulated Patients Utilizing the Radial Artery and Forearm Vein: A Two-Center Experience. *J Interv Cardiol.* 2006;*19*:258–63.

24. Yang CH, Guo GB, Yip HK. Bilateral Cardiac Catheterizations: The Safety and Feasibility of a Superficial Forearm Venous and Transradial Arterial Approach. *Int Heart J.* 2006;*47*:21–7.

25. Gilchrist IC, Moyer CD, Gascho JA. Transradial Right and Left Heart Catheterizations: A Comparison to Traditional Femoral Approach. *Catheter Cardiovasc Interv.* 2006;*67*:585–8.

Radial Access in Non-Cardiac Procedures

9

David Wells and James Davies

9.1 INTRODUCTION

Transradial access (TRA) for non-cardiac procedures is not new; however, it has taken some time for it to be implemented for non-cardiac procedures and for the industry to keep up with the appropriate size and length of equipment. There are many benefits to having this access option in the interventional radiology (IR) toolkit.

One of the key elements of this route is how comfortable it is for the patient compared to transfemoral access (TFA). There are no closure devices, and nothing is left behind. The target vessels are often easily accessed, and reliable hemostasis is a major benefit in patients with a high body mass index (BMI). In the day case setting, there is therefore added confidence to safe discharge, knowing there is almost no risk of access site complications. Often, there is a shorter patient recovery leading to immediate ambulation complementing the in-hours discharge policies of most interventional day case units [1–3].

TRA remains, however, an under-researched procedure within IR when compared to the large body of evidence in the cardiology literature. The largest single-centre experience documented 749 TRA (transradial access) procedures, finding no major access site complications and only a 0.5% crossover to TFA. Almost all patients (98%) who had undergone both TRA and TFA expressed a preference for the radial approach [4].

DOI: 10.1201/9781003153627-9

9.2 RADIAL ACCESS IN THE IR POPULATION

In many IR cases, longer sheaths and catheters are required to deliver the treatment options, and these can take between one hour to three hours to complete. It is rare that we need rapid radial access as most cases apart from trauma will be elective. Given these differences with respect to cardiology practice, it is important in IR to have a well-prepared vessel that is stabilised for cannulation and catheter manipulation to avoid the most common complications of vascular spasm and occlusion.

9.2.1 Vessel Preparation

To prepare the vessel for cannulation, 100 mcg (1 ml) Isoket is mixed with 9 ml 1% Lidocaine. Using USS guidance, the full 10 ml volume is infiltrated from a single needle puncture between the fascial layers of the radial artery at the wrist. This tumescence can be visualised with USS tracking 2–5 cm proximally around the radial artery. A microvascular access kit is then used to needle the artery with ultrasound, followed by the microwire and a 4F or 5F hydrophilic sheath.

9.2.2 Vessel Stabilisation

In a 20 ml luer lock syringe, a mixture of 2,000 IU heparin, 200 mcg Isoket, and 1.25 mg Verapamil is hemodiluted through the side arm of the sheath and slowly injected through the sheath into the forearm vessels. The combination of an anticoagulant, calcium antagonist and nitrate reduces the chances of vascular spasm and thrombosis and can be repeated if there are any issues with spasm throughout the procedure. This stabilises the forearm vessels for catheter and wire manipulation around the arch. In some procedures, deploying a longer sheath (e.g., 110 cm 5F hydrophilic sheath) into the distal aorta will aid in catheter manipulation whilst further minimising spasm risk.

9.2.3 Navigating to the Target Vessel

Once the radial artery is cannulated, it is common practice to advance an atraumatic wire with a 1.5 cm J tip and a hydrophilic coating. This avoids cannulating and traumatising the tiny side branches on the way to the subclavian artery (SCA). The left radial artery is by far the most common side for IR procedures as it eliminates crossing the arch vessels and the distance to the target vessel is reduced. Left-sided access requires the descending thoracic aorta to be negotiated.

With a type 1 arch, the left SCA is almost vertical, making cannulation of the descending thoracic aorta quite simple with a 4F multipurpose (MP) or a more angled 4F cobra catheter. In a type 2 or 3 arch, the left SCA is more acutely angled, and a reverse angle catheter, such as a 4F SIM 1 formed in the ascending thoracic aorta, is easily then negotiated into the descending aorta. If a longer sheath is needed for stability or to protect the artery from multiple catheter manipulations or exchanges, then it is advisable to take this over a long 300 cm 1.5 cm J tip wire into the descending aorta. Occasionally, the angle of the left subclavian origin will produce more tension on the equipment, and in this case, pushability can be problematic. Exchanging for a stiff or superstiff Amplatz wire, over which the sheath is advanced, can get around this problem.

9.3 VISCERAL AND RENAL

Radial access is an appealing alternative approach to the coeliac axis, mesenteric arteries and renal arteries. There are multiple treatment options for the different pathologies that are referred to IR for treatment. These vessels are often well aligned with equipment introduced from the left radial, with the push and torque from above often more favourable than from the femoral route below, where the sometimes-steep angle of the visceral arteries can increase overall tension within the platform, and therefore reduce stability in the target vessel. In settings where accurate placement of stents or coils is important, this can increase procedural risk, including non-target embolisation.

Coeliac axis angioplasty and stenting are possible using a combination of longer catheters and sheath sizes with angioplasty balloons and stents on longer 135 cm shafts. Many balloon-mounted stents will easily pass through a 5F 90–100 cm hydrophilic sheath over a 200–300 cm 0.018" or 0.014" wire. The splenic artery is also easily embolised from this position for both splenic trauma and treatment of aneurysms.

One of the most researched areas of TRA in IR is Transarterial Chemo-Embolisation (TACE) for liver tumours [5]. In this setting, high-dose chemoembolic agents are delivered directly into the vascular tumour mass, concentrating the chemotherapy within the liver. A similar treatment of selective internal radiotherapy (SIRT) is also available and has revolutionised the treatment of liver tumours, both primary and metastatic.

The renal arteries are easily accessed from above for angioplasty or stenting, for example, in the setting of renal artery stenosis with refractory hypertension. Stable renal trauma or renal tumours can be embolised and some renal artery aneurysms stented with covered stent grafts.

The inferior mesenteric artery gives rise to the superior rectal artery (SRA) and branches that are often the cause of hemorrhoidal bleeding refractory to traditional surgical treatments. Within the last decade, a novel approach to this has been in development, involving embolisation of the SRA branches with particles/coils or a combination. From a radial approach, patients can be admitted to a Radiology Day Case Unit (RDCU) and rapidly discharged.

9.4 PELVIC INTERVENTION

9.4.1 Uterine Fibroid Embolisation (UFE)

Radial access is particularly well-suited to UFE [6, 7], a procedure in which the patients are generally young women with heavy menstrual bleeding and pressure effects on the bladder from enlarged fibroids within the uterus. Patient comfort is an essential part of post-procedure care, especially the ability to mobilise immediately, and this opens the door to day case UFE [8].

With a 5F radial access and a 125 cm catheter, most uterine arteries (UAs) are easily cannulated, and it is simple to access both UAs by retracting the catheter into the distal aorta and cannulating the opposite side. Performing UFE can be a painful procedure, reproducing crampy menstrual-type pain. When TRA is used for UFE, after the embolisation, the patient can move around comfortably without the concern over groin access, significantly improving procedural tolerability. There is evidence that using this technique can reduce the time and radiation dose of the procedure to both the patient and operators [9].

9.4.2 Prostate Artery Embolisation (PAE)

Over the past decade, PAE has emerged as a minimally invasive treatment option for male patients suffering from lower urinary tract symptoms (LUTS) due to benign prostatic hyperplasia (BPH). More recently, the use of TRA to perform PAE has been described. Whilst technically challenging, the transradial technique offers several potential advantages in appropriately selected patients, which may improve the benefit-risk profile of PAE and improve

TABLE 9.1 Target vessel combinations for radial access; SMA superior mesenteric artery, IMA Inferior mesenteric artery, CIA common Iliac artery, EIA external iliac artery, IIA internal iliac artery, PAE prostate artery embolisation, UFE uterine fibroid embolisation, CFA common femoral artery, PF profunda femoris

VESSEL	SHEATH SIZE (FRENCH)	SHEATH LENGTH (CM)	PARENT CATHETER (CM)	MICRO CATHETER (CM)	WIRES (INCH)
Coeliac Axis	4-6F	90–100	100–125	130–150	0.035/0.018/0.014
SMA	4-6F	90–100	100–125	130–150	0.035/0.018/0.014
IMA	4-6F	90–100	100–125	130–150	0.035/0.018/0.014
Renal	4-6F	90–100	100–125	130–150	0.035/0.018/0.014
CIA	4-6F	≥110	125–150	150	0.035/0.018/0.014
EIA	4-6F	≥110	125–150	150	0.035/0.018/0.014
IIA	4-6F	≥110	125–150	150–175	0.035/0.018/0.014
PAE	5F	≥110	150	175	0.035/0.018/0.014
UFE	5F	≥110	125	150	0.035/0.018/0.014
CFA	4-6F	≥110	125–150	150	0.035/0.018/0.014
PF	4-6F	≥110	125–150	150–175	0.035/0.018/0.014

patient satisfaction [10, 11]. Radial access has become more workable recently with longer hydrophilic sheaths, longer parent catheters, and microcatheters (see Table 9.1). A stable radial platform consists of a 100–120 cm 4F hydrophilic sheath, 260–300 cm exchange wire, 4F 125–135 cm parent catheter, and 150–175 cm 1.9F microcatheters.

9.5 TRAUMA AND EMERGENCY

IR plays a critical role in the management of major trauma patients. Frequently, haemorrhage is due to solid organ injury, where the mechanism of injury, in the United Kingdom, is often high-impact blunt trauma. In these cases, the positioning of a pelvic binder can make femoral access challenging. In unstable patients where removal of the binder is contraindicated, having another arterial access option is important.

Major haemorrhage, whether that be traumatic or non-traumatic, can be complicated by several factors that affect clotting. The so-called lethal triad of coagulopathy, hypothermia, and acidosis, if left untreated, can lead to bleeding diatheses, where stopping the haemorrhage is the only way to get control. In these cases, femoral access also exposes the patient to additional risk, compounded by co-existing haemodynamic physiology. The radial approach provides a more accessible, controllable point of access if there is a complication. Although the evidence is limited, recent work has shown the safety and efficacy of TRA in trauma with non-inferiority over TFA and a lower complication profile [12].

Similarly, haemorrhage can often be confounded by, or caused by, the medication that the patient is receiving. Antiplatelet agents are commonplace, as are anticoagulants, and, increasingly, the use of new oral anticoagulants (NOACs). NOACs are less simple to reverse than traditional anticoagulants, such as warfarin. Again, in these cases, a radial approach should be considered [13]. The use of a radial approach in the emergency setting can be daunting for those not familiar with the technique, and certainly, the first time to use this access should not be in a bleeding patient where time is critical.

9.6 VASCULAR

9.6.1 Aortolliac Intervention

TRA should be considered in this setting if body habitus is not appropriate or there is a relative contraindication to TFA, such as a previous surgical groin or non-suitability for a closure device.

9.6.2 Iliac and Above Knee

The small size of the radial artery makes a 6 French sheath the maximum size recommended to limit the risk of radial artery occlusion or spasm. For aortoiliac disease, plain balloon angioplasty and bare metal stenting are possible, but covered stents and aortic interventions with stent grafts require larger sheaths and therefore, currently, an alternative access site. The use of large bore sheaths and delivery systems is increasingly common in cardiological practice (see Chapter 7). Adoption of these techniques into IR practice will expand the options for the use of larger systems. Radial access is an excellent choice for patients with femoral-femoral crossover graft problems where femoral access is not an option. It is also particularly useful in the common femoral artery and profunda femoris arteries in certain limb salvage situations where surgery is not feasible or appropriate for the patient and in threatened proximal graft stenoses in bypass grafts.

9.6.3 Below Knee

Unlike interventions from a femoral approach, stenting and drug-eluting technologies are not available in the lengths and diameters that radial access sheaths can accommodate in their present iterations. Below the knee intervention from the wrist is currently limited to angioplasty, and there are other limitations, such as the absence of re-entry devices and bail-out stents that are needed to improve the capabilities of TRA PAD interventions. A trans-pedal approach has been used by some IR operators in patients with limitations to TFA access.

9.7 NEUROVASCULAR INTERVENTION

Possibly one of the fastest growth areas in IR is in neurointervention, particularly with the rise of stroke thrombectomy, now the gold standard for ischaemic stroke in appropriately selected patients. These patients may well have had thrombolysis and are likely to be on antiplatelets and potentially other anticoagulation dependent on pre-existing cardiovascular risk. A recent study comparing TFA to TRA in patients undergoing thrombectomy following tissue plasminogen activator (TPA) demonstrated 12 vs. 0 access complications, respectively, with a shorter length of stay in the TRA group [14]. A similar complication profile was demonstrated in a further study in anterior circulation stroke, but most importantly, non-inferiority to TFA was demonstrated in terms of procedural time and first-pass reperfusion rate [15], providing encouraging data that quality is not sacrificed by TRA in these patients.

9.8 VESSEL CLOSURE

In common with cardiology practice, patent hemostasis addresses the balance between vessel wall closure and maintaining flow through the radial artery to avoid radial occlusion with the radial closure device. The catheters are withdrawn carefully over a wire to prevent the catheter tip from "dragging" on the wall of the artery. Patent haemostasis, as described in Chapter 6, can then be employed.

9.9 CONCLUSIONS

There is no doubt that the current evidence base for TRA in IR is limited in comparison with the cardiology data, but with increased acceptance and utilisation, this is beginning to change. TRA is a route of access that has unique advantages, and by following best practices and using a meticulous technique, operators can reap the benefits of a lower complication profile, improved patient safety, and improved patient experience. In the day case setting, TRA may improve productivity with shorter recovery and turnaround times.

REFERENCES

1. Wells RD. Ambulatory Care in Interventional Radiology: A Framework for Radiology Day-Case. *Clin Radiol*. doi: 10.1016/j.crad.2022.03.010
2. Roson N, Antolin A, Mast R, et al. Experience and Results After the Implementation of a Radiology Day Unit in a Reference Hospital. *Insights Imaging*. 2022;*13*:109. doi: 10.1186/s13244-022-01251-2
3. Lakshminarayan R, Bent C, Taylor J, Bryant T, Ahmad R, Diamantopoulos A, Morgan RA. Developing Day-Case Units: Imperative for Optimal Patient Care in Interventional Radiology. *Clin Radiol*. 2023 Apr;*78*(4):295–300. doi: 10.1016/j.crad.2022.11.017
4. Thakor AS, Alshammari MT, Liu DM, et al. Trans radial Access for Interventional Radiology: Single-Centre Procedural and Clinical Outcome Analysis. *Can Assoc Radiol J*. 2017;*68*(3):318–27. doi: 10.1016/j.carj.2016.09.003
5. Zhang, Xiaowu, et al. Trans Radial versus Transfemoral Access Without Closure Device for Trans Arterial Chemoembolization in Patients With Hepatocellular Carcinoma: A Randomized Trial. *Eur Radiol*. 2022;*32*(10):6812–19. doi: 10.1007/s00330-022-09038-1
6. Transradial Embolization, an Underused Type of Uterine Artery Embolization Approach: A Systematic Review Medicina (Kaunas). 2021 Feb;*57*(2):83. doi: 10.3390/medicina57020083
7. Nakhaei M, Mojtahedi A, Faintuch S, et al. Transradial and Transfemoral Uterine Fibroid Embolization Comparative Study: Technical and Clinical Outcomes. *J Vasc Interv Radiol*. 2020;*31*:123–9.
8. Wells RD, Allouni AK, Merron S. Uterine Fibroid Embolisation, Time for day case? The Stoke Protocol https://bads.co.uk/for-members/journal-of-one-day-surgery-jods/?id=1337#collapse2
9. Davies J, Allouni K, Wells D. Single-Centre Comparison of the Effect of Radial versus Femoral Access on Radiation Dose and Screening Time in Day Case Uterine Artery Embolisation. *J Daycase Surgery*. 2021 Nov;*31*(4).

10. Isaacson AJ, Fischman AM, Burke CT. Technical Feasibility of Prostatic Artery Embolization From a Transradial Approach. *AJR Am J Roentgenol.* 2016; *206*(2):442–4.

11. Bhatia S, Harward SH, Sinha VK, Narayanan G. Prostate Artery Embolization via Transradial or Transulnar versus Transfemoral Arterial Access: Technical Results. *J Vasc Interv Radiol.* 2017;*28*(6):898–905.

12. Adnan SM, Romagnonli AN, Elansary NN, Martinson JR, Madurska MJ, Dubose JJ, Scalea TM, Morrison JJ. Radial versus Femoral Arterial Access for Trauma Endovascular Interventions: A Noninferiority Study. *J Trauma Acute Care Surg.* 2020 Sep;*89*(3):458–63. doi: 10.1097/TA.0000000000002740

13. Titano JJ, Biederman DM, Zech J, et al. Safety and Outcomes of Trans Radial Access in Patients With International Normalized Ratio 1.5 or Above. *J Vasc Interv Radiol.* 2018;*29*(3):383–8. doi: 10.1016/j.jvir.2017.11.010

14. Catapano JS, Rumalla K, Farhadi DS, Parikh PP, Nguyen BA, Rutledge C, Srinivasan VM, Baranoski JF, Cole TS, Winkler EA, Desai SM. Safety and Efficacy of Radial Versus Femoral Artery Access for Mechanical Thrombectomy Procedures Following Intravenous Administration of Tissue Plasminogen Activator. *Stroke-Vasc Interv Neurol.* 2022 Sep;*2*(5):e000238.

15. Phillips TJ, Crockett MT, Selkirk GD, Kabra R, Chiu AH, Singh T, Phatouros C, McAuliffe W. Transradial versus Transfemoral Access for Anterior Circulation Mechanical Thrombectomy: Analysis of 375 Consecutive Cases. *Stroke Vasc Neurol.* 2021 Jun 1;*6*(2). doi: 10.1136/svn-2020-000624

Distal Radial Access

10

Karim Ratib and Darren Klass

10.1 INTRODUCTION

Distal radial or snuffbox access has been used more widely since 2017, following its description in a small subset of patients [1]. Prior to this, the technique had been used by a small number of cardiologists around the world, but data was not published in Western literature.

The increased use of social media, with cross-specialty collaboration and discussion around cases, promoted initially by Dr Kiemeneij, advanced the use of this technique much faster than conventional radial access and stimulated discussion on its use and validity as an alternative access site. This occurred at a time after significant growth in the use of conventional radial access for coronary interventions, as well as in interventional radiology, where there was increasing use for peripheral and neurological endovascular interventions. While neurological interventions use the right radial artery more than the left, due to the need for supra-aortic vessel cannulation, the left radial artery is used more commonly for peripheral interventions in interventional radiology. In coronary intervention, the left radial is frequently used for coronary bypass graft studies and to visualise left internal mammary grafts. Additionally, the left radial may offer simpler access and better support for coronary interventions, as brachiocephalic anatomy can be more tortuous and variable from the right compared to approaching via the left subclavian artery. Unfortunately, the other common reason for using the left radial is when the right radial has been found to be occluded. Access from the left wrist brings with it many challenges for the operator. Many angiography suites are designed for femoral intervention and

DOI: 10.1201/9781003153627-10

therefore patient positioning is such that the radiation protection is optimal from the right side of the patient, with little allowance made for working from the patient's left side. Additionally, if standing on the patient's left side, the position of the operator's dominant hand is switched, which alters the ergonomics of the procedure significantly compared to the more familiar manipulations from the right side of the patient. An alternative is staying on the right side and bringing the patient's left wrist across their body to allow for puncture, with the left wrist in a similar position to the left groin. While this solves some of the issues, having the patient's arm in this position, supinated for extended periods, can be uncomfortable for the patient. Distal access provides an alternative solution for many of these challenges faced with left radial access, in addition to potential clinical advantages, which will be discussed throughout this chapter.

10.2 ANATOMY

The distal radial artery forms the only content of the anatomical snuffbox. It is bordered by the extensor pollicus longus and brevis and abductor pollicus tendons, the floor is made up of the scaphoid and trapezium, and the roof is comprised of branches of the superficial radial nerve and the cephalic vein. This anatomy can prove challenging for puncture. Some of these challenges are reduced with experience, and some are much easier to address with the use of ultrasound.

1. The optimal site for puncture of the distal radial is a shorter length of vessel than that in conventional radial access; thus, the margin for error in selecting the puncture site is reduced. The vessel should be accessed in the snuffbox over the scaphoid or trapezium to facilitate haemostasis with compression. The more distal vessel, although palpable in the interosseous space of the thumb and index finger, is less desirable for access, as there are no bones to provide support for haemostasis, which may increase the risk of bleeding.
2. Depending on the site of access, the tendons which form the borders of the snuffbox may be superficial to the distal radial artery, and failure to identify these tendons at the time of puncture may lead to pain during the procedure and tendonitis post-procedure.
3. The distal radial artery is smaller than the artery in the conventional access site [2–5], and although not clinically significant, this does increase the complexity of access, particularly if palpation is used. Utilising ultrasound for access improves access rates and decreases the incidence of haematomas [6].

4. The vessel traverses the anatomical snuffbox from medial to lateral, which makes access more challenging than conventional access. Access and subsequent blood from the needle do not ensure reliable passage of the wire. Elderly patients, particularly females, are prone to osteoarthritis in the thumb carpometacarpal joint, with osteophyte formation that may complicate the course further. Again, the use of ultrasound may help with identifying the course of the artery and help direct the passage of the wire.

5. The margin for error is less in the snuffbox than with conventional access. The vessel is superficial, and therefore a small haematoma can compress the vessel enough to make it extremely difficult to access. The success of access decreases with repeated attempts due to haematoma formation, focal dissection, or a focal intramural haematoma, all of which can be identified with ultrasound.

6. The periosteum of the underlying carpal bones is extremely sensitive, and contact with the needle causes discomfort for the patient. Single wall puncture, although never shown to be safer than double wall puncture, should minimise this risk.

The anatomical advantages, however, are the greatest benefit of this access site. Because the vessel is so superficial, haemostasis can be much shorter than conventional access with resultant lower rates of radial artery occlusion (RAO) [2] both at the distal puncture site and more proximal at the conventional radial site (which can still be injured by the passage of wires or sheath despite not being punctured). Nevertheless, avoiding puncture and compression at the conventional radial site may reduce injury to this part of the artery, preserving this vessel for future use for intervention or for dialysis fistulae or coronary bypass grafts.

The distal radial artery gives origin to the superficial palmar branch, which is variable in its location but is often proximal to the snuffbox, thus providing an early branch point in the vessel. This provides a significant anatomical advantage as if a radial artery occlusion should occur at the distal puncture site; the occlusion will often stop at this branch point, allowing only a short segment occlusion, preserving the conventional radial artery for future use or access.

10.3 ULTRASOUND-GUIDED ACCESS

With many of the challenges due to the anatomy, ultrasound-guided access provides a much more predictable method of safe access compared to palpation alone. Ultrasound easily identifies variations in anatomy, tortuosity, and

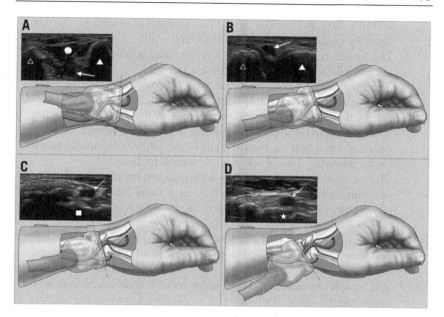

FIGURE 10.1 Ultrasound and anatomic correlation. (A) – (D) Different transducer positions and their corresponding ultrasound images starting distally at the first dorsal web space (A), moving proximally to the anatomical snuffbox over the scaphoid (D). Arrow: Distal radial artery; circle: First dorsal interosseous muscle; filled triangle: Thumb metacarpal; unfilled triangle: Index metacarpal; square: Trapezium bone; star: Scaphoid bone.

Adapted from Hadjivassiliou A, Kiemeneij F, Nathan S, Klass D. Ultrasound-Guided Access to the Distal Radial Artery at the Anatomical Snuffbox for Catheter-Based Vascular Interventions: A Technical Guide. *EuroIntervention.* 2021 Mar 19;16(16):1342–1348. doi: 10.4244/EIJ-D-19-00555. PMID: 31380781; PMCID: PMC9724968.

vessel size and allows for optimal puncture (Figure 10.1). This technique is used as a standard in interventional radiology but is more sporadic in cardiology and neuroradiology; for this reason, some background into the techniques and tips for successful access are essential.

1. Utilising ultrasound ensures the vessel is punctured over the trapezium or scaphoid, thus providing reliable support for haemostasis.
2. Blind puncture increases the risk of access through one of the tendons, forming a border of the snuffbox. This is not only painful for the patient during the procedure but can cause tendonitis post-procedure.

Identification and avoidance of these tendons is essential, and this can only be done reliably with ultrasound.

3. The vessel is smaller than the conventional access site. Utilising ultrasound for access improves access rates [6].

4. The more complex route of the vessel through the snuffbox can make wire advancement difficult with needle access in the vessel due to the needle being against the wall of the vessel. Evaluation with ultrasound will demonstrate the path of the vessel, and the operator can adjust the insertion site or direction of the needle based on the anatomy. This is not possible with palpation.

5. The success of access decreases with repeated attempts due to haematoma formation, focal dissection, or a focal intramural haematoma. Ultrasound has been shown to decrease the number of attempts required and thus lower rates of failure [6].

6. Avoiding contact with the periosteum with the needle is preferable, and this is easily achieved with a single wall, ultrasound-guided puncture.

7. The complexity of access overall is greater with distal access than with conventional access. Utilisation of ultrasound improves the success rate of access and decreases conversion to conventional access [7].

10.4 PATIENT SET-UP

One of the many advantages of this technique is the ability to position the patient with many different options, depending on the side of access, operator preference, and procedure.

For right-sided access, the positioning and preparation of the patient and wrist do not change significantly from conventional access; however, with distal access, the patient's forearm can be held in pronation for the procedure, which is more comfortable and decreases the patient's propensity to move the hand during the procedure due to discomfort.

For left-sided access, the patient can be positioned as for a right-sided puncture, but the arm is adducted across the patient's body to allow for access to the distal radial artery with the wrist positioned over the patient's groin. This improves the operator's ergonomic position and allows the forearm to remain in pronation, which is more comfortable for the patient. Various techniques can be employed to keep the wrist in this position, including a commercially available support which holds the patient's arm in position.

A further option for operators, if the suite is versatile enough to allow, the operator can stand on the patient's left side with the arm abducted 45°–90°, and the procedure can be performed with the operator in this position, which in addition decreases the operator's radiation exposure, as there is increased distance from the radiation source. This set-up is used more widely in interventional radiology, where left-sided access is used in the majority of procedures. This technique has been shown to decrease the operators' radiation exposure [8].

The advantage of placing the arm away from the patient is also used more widely in interventional radiology, as most procedures are performed in the abdomen and pelvis (oncology, uterine and prostate embolisation). Placing the arm across the body can, in certain patients, cause the arm to remain in the desired field of view.

10.5 DISTAL RADIAL ACCESS FOR PERIPHERAL INTERVENTION

The use of distal radial access is now well described in the literature. The implementation in visceral, peripheral, and neuro-intervention has only been described more commonly in the last ten years. One of the likely driving forces for distal radial access gaining increased use is due to endovascular specialties using this technique with an increase in the published literature on the subject.

Many procedures have much more favourable ergonomics from the wrist. All the visceral and pelvic vessels extend in a caudal direction, making cannulation much easier and more stable with access from above. The faster haemostasis achieved with distal access allows patients to ambulate immediately post-procedure and thus decreases hospital stay [2]. For many patients undergoing oncological interventions, providing an alternative access site with a shorter observation period and, thus, discharge post-procedure can have a significant impact on patient quality of life. Radial access has been shown to decrease radiation exposure to both operator and patient in oncology interventions [8] and in prostate and fibroid embolisation [9, 10]. The use of distal radial access in the neuro-interventional space has probably increased proportionally more than either body or coronary interventions, as many operators transitioning from femoral to radial make the transition directly to distal radial access [11].

10.6 DISTAL RADIAL ACCESS FOR CORONARY INTERVENTION

In the coronary field, distal radial has been used as an alternative to conventional radial and can be used across a broad range of procedures, including complex percutaneous coronary intervention (PCI) using larger-bore sheaths (7F), as well as sheathless access with large-bore catheters. The largest, multi-centre, randomised trial, comparing distal to conventional radial for coronary angiography and angioplasty [12], included 1,309 patients. The investigators found no difference in the primary end point of forearm radial occlusion as detected by pre-discharge ultrasound. Crossover rates were higher for distal radial, as was time to arterial access and radial artery spasm. These findings are likely to be related to the learning curve, as well as the smaller calibre of the more distal artery. There were no differences in vascular complications, but haemostasis times were significantly lower with distal radial, with a mean reduction of over 30 minutes compared to conventional radial access. It should be noted that the radial artery occlusion rates were very low in both arms of the study (<1%) using optimal haemostasis in the conventional radial group with patent haemostasis. Similar results were achieved with distal radial while using a much simpler, less labour-intensive haemostasis protocol with simple compression techniques.

A meta-analysis, including 28 randomised studies of conventional to distal radial, with over 9,000 patients [13], have shown similar results but additionally observed a reduction in the incidence of forearm radial occlusion when distal radial access is used. A detailed study of hand function [14] following distal radial access did not find any adverse effects.

10.7 CONCLUSIONS

Overall, distal radial artery access is safe and allows for a wide range of diagnostic and interventional procedures. It is associated with simpler and shorter haemostasis at the expense of higher initial crossover rates. This makes distal radial access attractive, especially in an overburdened health-care system where there may be limited resources to optimally manage post-procedural haemostasis. Ultrasound guidance may shorten the learning curve and reduce the crossover rate.

REFERENCES

1. Kiemeneij F. Left Distal Transradial Access in the Anatomical Snuffbox for Coronary Angiography (ldTRA) and Interventions (ldTRI). *EuroIntervention.* 2017 Sep 20;*13*(7):851–7. doi: 10.4244/EIJ-D-17-00079

2. Hadjivassiliou A, Cardarelli-Leite L, Jalal S, Chung J, Liu D, Ho S, Klass D. Left Distal Transradial Access (ldTRA): A Comparative Assessment of Conventional and Distal Radial Artery Size. *Cardiovasc Intervent Radiol.* 2020 Jun;*43*(6):850–7. doi: 10.1007/s00270-020-02485-7

3. Li SS, Li JM, Liu LL, Liu W, Yang H, Feng CG. Analysis of the Risk Factors Related to the Success Rate of Distal Transradial Artery Access in Patients with Coronary Heart Disease. *Risk Manag Healthc Policy.* 2022 Apr 13;*15*:657–63. doi: 10.2147/RMHP.S357780

4. Lee JW, Son JW, Go TH, Kang DR, Lee SJ, Kim SE, Cho DH, Park YJ, Youn YJ, Ahn MS, Ahn SG, Kim JY, Yoo BS, Yoon J, Lee SH. Reference Diameter and Characteristics of the Distal Radial Artery Based on Ultrasonographic Assessment. *Korean J Intern Med.* 2022 Jan;*37*(1):109–18. doi: 10.3904/kjim.2020.685

5. Deora S, Sharma SK, Choudhary R, Kaushik A, Garg PK, Khera PS, Singh K, Shah S, Patel TM. Assessment and Comparison of Distal Radial Artery Diameter in Anatomical Snuff Box With Conventional Radial Artery Before Coronary Catheterization. *Indian Heart J.* 2022 Jul-Aug;*74*(4):322–6. doi: 10.1016/j.ihj.2022.06.007

6. Nguyen P, Makris A, Hennessy A, Jayanti S, Wang A, Park K, Chen V, Nguyen T, Lo S, Xuan W, Leung M, Juergens C. Standard versus Ultrasound-Guided Radial and Femoral Access in Coronary Angiography and Intervention (SURF): A Randomised Controlled Trial. *EuroIntervention.* 2019 Aug 9;*15*(6):e522–30. doi: 10.4244/EIJ-D-19-00336

7. Maitra S, Baidya DK, Ray BR, Chowhan G, Bhattacharjee S. Comparison of Ultrasound Guided Dorsal Radial Artery Cannulation and Conventional Radial Artery Cannulation at the Volar Aspect of Wrist: A Pilot Randomized Controlled Trial. *J Vasc Access.* 2022 Apr 26. doi: 10.1177/11297298221093953

8. Yamada R, Bracewell S, Bassaco B, Camacho J, Anderson MB, Conrad A, Lynn C, Burns P, Collins H, Guimaraes M. Transradial Versus Transfemoral Arterial Access in Liver Cancer Embolization: Randomized Trial to Assess Patient Satisfaction. *J Vasc Interv Radiol.* 2018 Jan;*29*(1):38–43. doi: 10.1016/j.jvir.2017.08.024

9. Bhatia S, Harward SH, Sinha VK, Narayanan G. Prostate Artery Embolization via Transradial or Transulnar versus Transfemoral Arterial Access: Technical Results. *J Vasc Interv Radiol.* 2017 Jun;*28*(6):898–905. doi: 10.1016/j.jvir.2017.02.029

10. Mortensen C, Chung J, Liu D, Ho S, Legiehn G, Machan L, Klass D. Prospective Study on Total Fluoroscopic Time in Patients Undergoing Uterine Artery Embolization: Comparing Transradial and Transfemoral Approaches. *Cardiovasc Intervent Radiol.* 2019 Mar;*42*(3):441–7. doi: 10.1007/s00270-018-2100-3

11. Kühn AL, de Macedo RK, Singh J, Massari F, Puri AS. Distal Radial Access in the Anatomical Snuffbox for Neurointerventions: A Feasibility, Safety, and Proof-of-Concept Study. *J Neurointerv Surg.* 2020 Aug;*12*(8):798–801. doi: 10.1136/neurintsurg-2019-015604

12. Aminian A, Sgueglia GA, Wiemer M, Kefer J, Gasparini GL, Ruzsa Z, van Leeuwen MAH, Ungureanu C, Leibundgut G, Vandeloo B, Kedev S, Bernat I, Ratib K, Iglesias JF, Al Hage E, Posteraro GA, Pascut D, Maes F, Regazzoli D, Kakonyi K, Meijers TA, Colletti G, Krivoshei L, Lochy S, Zafirovska B, Horák D, Nolan J, Degrauwe S, Tobita K, Saito S. Distal Versus Conventional Radial Access for Coronary Angiography and Intervention: The DISCO RADIAL Trial. *JACC Cardiovasc Interv.* 2022 Jun 27;*15*(12):1191–1201. doi: 10.1016/j.jcin.2022.04.032

13. Feghaly J, Chen K, Blanco A, Pineda AM. Distal versus Conventional Radial Artery Access for Coronary Catheterization: A Systematic Review and Meta-Analysis. *Catheter Cardiovasc Interv.* 2023 Mar;*101*(4):722–36. doi: 10.1002/ccd.30602

14. Sgueglia GA, Hassan A, Harb S, Ford TJ, Koliastasis L, Milkas A, Zappi DM, Navarro Lecaro A, Ionescu E, Rankin S, Said CF, Kuiper B, Kiemeneij F. International Hand Function Study Following Distal Radial Access: The RATATOUILLE Study. *JACC Cardiovasc Interv.* 2022 Jun 27;*15*(12):1205–15. doi: 10.1016/j.jcin.2022.04.023

Alternative Access Sites

11

Bing Wei Thaddeus Soh, Eoin Fahy, Thomas Kiernan and Samer Arnous

11.1 INTRODUCTION

While transradial access remains the default approach, alternative access sites should be considered in situations encountering challenging anatomical variants (radial loops, tortuosity, and high take-off), non-palpable radial arteries, radial artery vasospasm, or where large-bore access is required. Crossover to the contralateral left radial artery should be considered before crossover to transfemoral access due to improved safety, quality of life, and cost-effectiveness of transradial compared to transfemoral access [1, 2]. Furthermore, transulnar has been shown to be non-inferior to transradial access and therefore should also be considered before attempting crossover to the transfemoral approach [3–5]. However, transfemoral access remains an important alternative access site for procedures performed within the catheter laboratory [6, 7], and all interventionalists should retain proficiency in the technique to reduce the risk of complications in situations where its use is mandated [8]. As a last resort, transbrachial access can be performed either percutaneously or via arterial cutdown to the brachial artery if other access options are not available [9–11].

DOI: 10.1201/9781003153627-11

11.2 LEFT RADIAL ACCESS

Right radial artery access remains the default approach in many centres for most cases. Despite this, the left radial artery approach confers several advantages. Meta-analysis comparing coronary procedures performed via left- and right-transradial access has shown a small but significant reduction in fluoroscopy time and contrast use favouring left radial access, without a difference in the access failure rate [12]. These advantages are explained by favourable left radial artery anatomical features such as reduced incidence of subclavian tortuosity and only one level of bifurcation to be traversed since the left subclavian artery arises directly from the aortic arch. The straighter route to the coronaries from the left translates to easier catheter manipulation and coronary engagement when compared to the more complex S-shaped geometry of the subclavian-innominate-aorta axis when accessing via the right side. Graft studies are also more easily performed from the left due to a more direct, coaxial approach to the left internal mammary artery and saphenous vein grafts.

Despite these advantages, the right radial remains the default approach predominantly because of the ergonomic difficulties of performing prolonged procedures on a partially pronated left hand draped across the abdomen with further limitations in obese patients. The left radial approach should therefore be considered in patients with expected subclavian tortuosity (age ≥ 75 years old, short stature), concomitant graft studies to be performed, and after failed access via the right radial artery. Set-up for left radial access may commence once the patient is comfortable on the catheterisation laboratory table. To cannulate the left radial artery, operators may choose to remain to the patient's right and lean across the patient while bringing the patient's arm across the abdomen (Figure 11.1), or they may move to the left of the patient. If they choose the latter, a modified set-up (Figure 11.2) can be used where a left radial board is placed beneath the left arm to support the wrist at 90 degrees abduction. A soft roll is placed under the left wrist in supination to allow access to the left radial puncture site. Conscious sedation and local anaesthetic are administered to mitigate arterial vasospasm. The left radial artery is punctured with the standard or modified Seldinger technique. After successful cannulation, a 0.018″ guidewire is inserted, over which a sheath with dilator is advanced. A "radial cocktail" containing anticoagulation (2,500 to 5,000 units of heparin) and vasodilators (nitroglycerin, verapamil, or nicardipine) is administered through the sheath to mitigate arterial vasospasm and occlusion. The left hand is then moved into position by lifting off the radial board and bringing the arm across the abdomen in partial pronation. The arm can be secured in this position with a sling to fix the hand in place. The operator performs the rest of the procedure from the right side of the table. If difficult

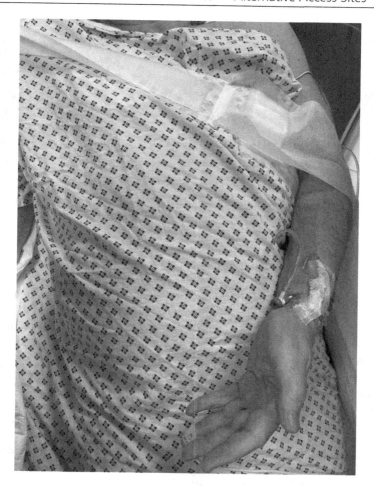

FIGURE 11.1 Adducting the left arm across the patients abdomen allows puncture while standing to the right of the patient. Use of a sling or support under the elbow helps maintain position during the procedure.

catheter manipulation is anticipated/encountered from resistance caused by vasospasm or challenging anatomical variants, several strategies could be attempted to overcome this: using hydrophilic-coated and smaller-calibre sheaths, taking radial angiography to confirm patency or challenging anatomy (loops, tortuosity), using hydrophilic guidewires (Silverway–Asahi, Radifocus–Terumo) to negotiate and cross complex arterial anatomy, and employing balloon or catheter-assisted tracking techniques to smoothly track catheters through tortuous segments.

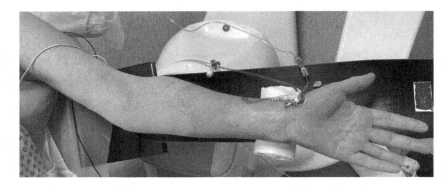

FIGURE 11.2   Patients arm in abduction on an arm board and supported at the wrist allows puncture from the left side of the table.

Standard Judkins left and right catheters (JR4, JL3.5) can be used to effectively cannulate the coronary ostia as their orientation within the ascending aorta is similar to that of catheters inserted via femoral access. For graft studies, Judkins right catheter (JR4) may be used for engaging the left internal mammary artery and saphenous vein grafts on the anterior surface of the aorta, but specific coronary bypass catheters, Amplatz left and internal mammary (IM) catheters (Bartorelli-Cozzi) may be considered depending on the anatomy. After the procedure, the sheath is removed, and patent haemostasis is achieved by using a pulse oximeter sensor. By confirming radial artery patency by detecting the presence of a plethysmographic signal, the risk of radial artery occlusion is reduced by preventing total occlusion and thrombosis during haemostasis. As with the right radial approach, radial artery vasospasm and radial artery occlusion remain its biggest limitation. With the overall incidence of radial artery occlusion reported at 7.7% (up to 38% reported in some studies), mitigating techniques (heparin, patent haemostasis) remain important as high-dose heparin (5,000 IU compared with 2,000 to 3,000 IU) have been shown to reduce occlusion rates from 10.5% to 4.4%, while patent haemostasis has shown reductions from 10% to 1.4% [13, 14].

11.3 ULNAR ACCESS

Arising from the brachial artery below the elbow, the ulnar artery is an alternative forearm access site. It extends distally along the medial aspect of the forearm accompanied by the ulnar nerve medially adjacent to it. Compared to the radial artery, the ulnar artery may have a larger diameter and is less prone to vasospasm due to fewer alpha-adrenergic receptors [15]. Despite favourable characteristics, transulnar access is still infrequently and non-routinely used due to its relative depth and proximity to the ulnar nerve [16]. The ulnar artery runs deeper than the radial artery; hence, it is less readily palpable and more difficult to access without ultrasound guidance. Despite technical difficulties, several meta-analyses have demonstrated similar efficacy between transulnar and transradial access [3–5]. Access-site complication rates (arterial occlusion, haematoma formation, and pseudo aneurysm) were similar between transulnar and transradial access, with subgroup analysis demonstrating a lower risk of local bleeding (4.9% vs. 8.5%, OR 0.55, 95% CI [0.33, 0.93]; $P = 0.02$) when transulnar access was used for percutaneous coronary intervention (PCI) [5].

The safety and feasibility of transulnar access in the setting of ipsilateral radial artery occlusion have also been investigated with no reported difference in major vascular complications or hand ischaemia rates when compared to patients with patent radial arteries, although the studies of this approach are numerically small with limited duration of follow-up [17]. Guideline documents caution against this approach, and careful consideration of all access options is needed before performing simultaneous ipsilateral radial and ulnar canulation or ulnar canulation in the setting of a known radial occlusion.

With equivalent safety and efficacy profile, the transulnar approach is an important alternative access site which should be considered when radial access is not possible (unfavourable anatomical variant, occlusion, vasospasm) or in those with alternative uses for radial arteries (grafts for bypass, fistula for haemodialysis access).

Set-up for right transulnar access is positionally similar to right radial access. A radial board is placed beneath the right arm to support the wrist positioned beside the body. The right wrist is hyperextended in supination with a soft roll beneath. Conscious sedation and local anaesthetic are administered in the same fashion for the same purpose (mitigate arterial vasospasm). The ulnar artery is palpated proximal to the pisiform bone using the proximal medial wrist crease as the surface landmark. If not palpable, an attempt to identify the deep ulnar artery should be performed under ultrasound guidance. The ulnar artery should be punctured from a lateral approach to avoid trauma to the ulnar nerve and flexor carpi ulnaris. A sheath is advanced in the same fashion after successful cannulation, and a "radial cocktail" is administered for the same purpose. The rest of the procedure is performed with a conventional radial approach.

At the end of the procedure, the sheath is removed, and haemostasis is achieved with a conventional compression device applied over the ulnar artery puncture site. While the incidence of ulnar artery vasospasm is low (fewer adrenergic receptors), ulnar artery occlusion rates of up to 11.9% have been reported [14]. Despite this reported rate, we do not recommend adopting patent haemostasis techniques for ulnar cases – as the artery does not directly overly bone, it is more difficult to reliably compress with an increased potential for haematoma formation from attempted patent techniques – compression should be applied and maintained until haemostasis is secure.

11.4 FEMORAL ACCESS

The femoral artery was historically considered the default approach for cardiac catheterisation and still remains the most popular access site in the United States [6, 7]. Compared to transradial approach, the transfemoral approach is associated with a greater risk of access-site complications, prolonged hospitalisation, and mortality [2]. Yet despite its effectiveness, the use of the transradial approach is limited by its Achilles heel: radial artery vasospasm, reported to occur in up to 30% of cases, is the most common cause of procedural failure and radial artery occlusion [18, 19]. Radial artery occlusion, the commonest post-procedural complication of the transradial approach (reported overall incidence of 7.7%), has great clinical implications as it prohibits future access via transradial approach and radial artery utilisation for grafts or fistula construction [13, 20]. The transfemoral approach, therefore, remains an important alternative access site for situations where forearm approaches have failed or when large-bore access is required. Its extensive history of use, lower likelihood for arterial vasospasm, and greater propensity for patency make this approach a core skill within the catheterisation laboratory which all interventionalists should be adequately trained in to minimise access-site complications when compelled to use it [8].

To mitigate bleeding and access-site complications, contemporary transfemoral access techniques involve clinical assessment, imaging guidance, micropuncture technique, femoral angiography, and vascular closure devices. The clinical assessment focuses on identifying patients with unfavourable characteristics: such as patients with severe peripheral artery disease (claudication, ulcers, gangrene, previous vascular interventions), morbid obesity, profound orthopnoea, or on oral anticoagulation (warfarin with INR $\geq$ 2.0, rivaroxaban, apixaban, edoxaban, and dabigatran). To minimise access-site complications, fluoroscopic and ultrasound imaging play a vital role in localising the ideal femoral artery puncture site: the common femoral artery over the femoral head, above the common femoral bifurcation, and below the inguinal ligament. The middle horizontal margin and lower horizontal margin of the femoral head are established fluoroscopic landmarks that correspond to 98.5% or 77% of patients, respectively, having femoral bifurcation at or below this line, thus guiding operators away from "low stick" punctures [21]. Ultrasound imaging allows real-time visualisation of the common femoral artery and bifurcation into the superficial femoral artery and profunda femoris and should be considered for all transfemoral procedures. This allows identification of unfavourable anatomy (calcific plaques, high bifurcations), operator flexibility in access site (common femoral or superficial femoral artery), and direct visualisation of advancing the micropuncture needle. Compared to fluoroscopy, ultrasound guidance has been shown to reduce the number of cannulation attempts, time to access, venepuncture risk, and access-site complications [22]. The micropuncture technique employs a 21-gauge echogenic micropuncture needle with a 0.018″ guidewire, resulting in smaller arteriotomy sites [23].

Set-up for transfemoral access requires the patients to be comfortable in a supine position on the catheterisation laboratory table. The groin region is exposed while preserving dignity, and the right femoral pulse is palpated at the right femoral crease. Local anaesthetic is administered over this region to ensure patient comfort. A 21-gauge micropuncture needle is used to penetrate the skin under real-time ultrasound guidance (Figure 11.3a) and puncture the common femoral artery above the bifurcation (Figures 11.3b–d). After successful cannulation, a 0.018″ guidewire is advanced under fluoroscopic guidance to ensure it follows the route of the external iliac artery. The femoral sheath with dilator is advanced over the guidewire, and a femoral arteriogram is performed by injecting contrast through the sheath to confirm adequate positioning.

At the end of the procedure, the femoral sheath should be removed as early as possible to reduce vascular complications. The sheath should be removed immediately in diagnostic procedures if no anticoagulation was used. Where intraprocedural anticoagulation was used, the sheath should be removed with the application of a vascular closure device (AngioSeal, ProGlide) or alternatively when the anticoagulation has been reversed over time (activated clotting time < 150–160 seconds or 6–8 hours after the last dose of enoxaparin). After sheath removal, haemostasis is achieved using manual compression applied with three fingers proximal to the site of the skin puncture. The duration of compression is loosely determined by the sheath size where a general rule of five minutes per French size is followed. Several active and passive vascular closure devices have been developed to accelerate the haemostasis process, but a discussion of their efficacy and use is beyond the scope of this chapter (Figure 11.4).

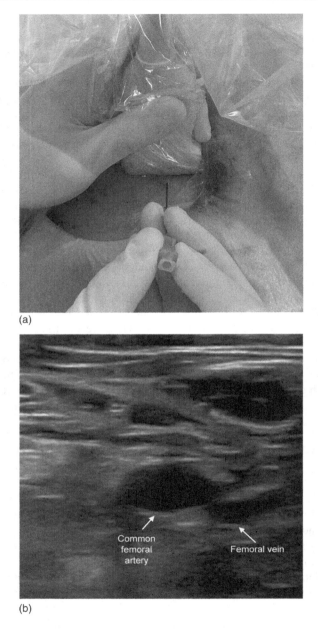

(a)

(b)

FIGURE 11.3 (a) Ultrasound-guided femoral puncture (short axis, out of plane puncture), (b) ultrasound short access view of common femoral artery and partially compressed femoral vein.

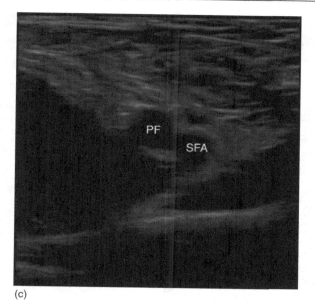

(c)

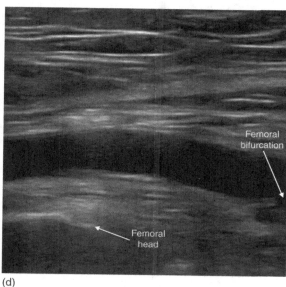

(d)

FIGURE 11.3 (Continued)   (c) short access view below the femoral bifurcation, demonstrating the superficial femoral artery (SFA) and profunda femoris (PF), (d) long axis view of the common femoral artery can help identify the femoral head.

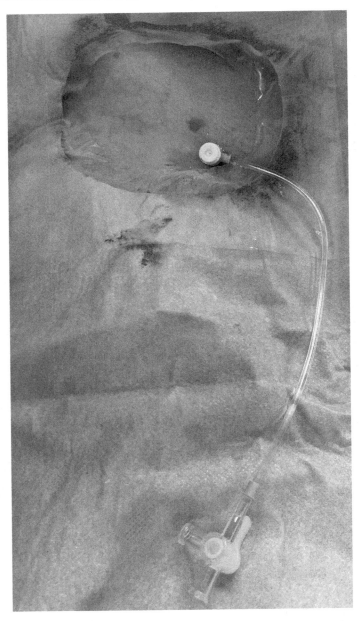

FIGURE 11.4 Successful vascular access: A close-up view of the surface anatomy following the successful insertion of a 6-French femoral sheath into the right common femoral artery.

11.5 BRACHIAL ACCESS

Gaining access via the brachial artery was originally performed by Sones using an arterial cutdown technique exposing the brachial artery [9]. Despite advances permitting percutaneous brachial puncture, operators have been swayed towards transradial or transfemoral approaches due to historically high complication rates using the transbrachial approach [10, 24]. As the main artery descends down the upper limb accompanied by the median nerve, the brachial artery is susceptible to serious vascular and upper limb neurological complications [11]. With clear advantages from the transradial approach, there are limited randomised studies evaluating the use of the transbrachial approach. Pooled data from one randomised controlled trial and five observational studies suggest that the transbrachial approach has lower bleeding complications compared to the transfemoral approach, but the evidence base supporting this remains poor [25]. However, recent case reports of administering mechanical circulatory support through transbrachial instead of the conventional transfemoral approach could potentially develop new interest in this access site in the future [26].

The set-up for the transbrachial approach is positionally similar to right radial access. A radial board is placed beneath the right arm to support a fully extended arm with the right hand in supination. The brachial artery is palpated proximally in the right antecubital fossa. Conscious sedation is administered as convention, and local anaesthetic is applied to the overlying tissue. A surgical cutdown approach should only be employed by an operator who has extensive previous experience of this technique – in the absence of a cardiologist with suitable training, a vascular surgeon should be consulted to provide assistance with securing safe and secure surgical access.

The brachial artery can be accessed via percutaneous puncture – interventional radiologists are frequently skilled in this access technique and should be consulted for assistance where possible. Under ultrasound guidance, the brachial artery is punctured on the anterior surface with a 21-gauge micropuncture needle, followed by advancing a sheath over an inserted 0.018-inch guidewire. Heparin is administered after sheath insertion to minimise thrombotic complications. At the end of the procedure, the brachial sheath should be removed as soon as anticoagulation has worn off or been corrected. Like femoral access, haemostasis is most commonly achieved through manual compression, but vascular closure devices may be considered. The arm is then placed in a sling for 24 hours.

11.6 CONCLUSION

Where right-transradial access is not possible, an alternative access site must be obtained. We described the left-transradial, transulnar, transfemoral, and brachial approaches as potential alternative sites used in contemporary practice for gaining access to cardiac catheterisation. Both left-transradial and the transulnar approaches have shown equal safety and efficacy compared to conventional right-transradial access and should be considered. Where large-bore access is required or when forearm approaches have failed, the transfemoral approach should be considered. Transbrachial access is not routinely used, and few cardiologists have sufficient experience in this approach. Brachial access should only be considered as a last resort and with the support and aid of interventional radiologists or vascular surgeons.

REFERENCES

1. Ferrante G. Radial versus Femoral Access for Coronary Interventions Across the Entire Spectrum of Patients With Coronary Artery Disease: A Meta-Analysis of Randomized Trials. *J Am Coll Cardiol Intv.* 2016;*9*(14):1419–34.
2. Kolkailah AA. Transradial versus Transfemoral Approach for Diagnostic Coronary Angiography and Percutaneous Coronary Intervention in People With Coronary Artery Disease. *Cochrane Database Syst Rev.* 2018;*4*. https://doi.org/10.1002/14651858.CD012318.pub2
3. Dahal K. Transulnar versus Transradial Access for Coronary Angiography or Percutaneous Coronary Intervention: A Meta-Analysis of Randomized Controlled Trials. *Catheter Cardiovasc Interv.* 2016;*87*(5):857–65.
4. Fernandez R. Safety and Efficacy of Ulnar Artery Approach for Percutaneous Cardiac Catheterization: Systematic Review and Meta-Analysis. *Catheter Cardiovasc Interv.* 2018;*91*(7):1273–80.
5. Sedhom R. Transulnar versus Transradial Access for Coronary Angiography and Percutaneous Coronary Intervention: A Meta-Analysis of Randomized Controlled Trials. *Cardiovasc Revasc Med.* 2021;*26*:39–45.
6. Rao SV. Trends in the Prevalence and Outcomes of Radial and Femoral Approaches to Percutaneous Coronary Intervention: A Report From the National Cardiovascular Data Registry. *J Am Coll Cardiol Intv.* 2008;*1*(4):379–86.
7. Feldman DN. Adoption of Radial Access and Comparison of Outcomes to Femoral Access in Percutaneous Coronary Intervention: An Updated Report From the National Cardiovascular Data Registry (2007–2012). *Circulation.* 2013;*127*(23):2295–306.

8. Azzalini L. The Benefits Conferred by Radial Access for Cardiac Catheterization Are Offset by a Paradoxical Increase in the Rate of Vascular Access Site Complications With Femoral Access: The Campeau Radial Paradox. *J Am Coll Cardiol Intv.* 2015;*8*(14):1854–64.

9. Sones FM. Cine Coronary Arteriography. *Mod Concepts Cardiovasc Dis.* 1962;*31*:735–8.

10. Fergusson DJ. Percutaneous Entry of the Brachial Artery for Left Heart Catheterization Using a Sheath. *Cathet Cardiovasc Diagn.* 1981;*7*(1):111–14.

11. Protty M. Brachial Arterial Access for PCI: An Analysis of the British Cardiovascular Intervention Society Database. *EuroIntervention.* 2022;*17*(13): 1100–3.

12. Shah RM. Comparison of Transradial Coronary Procedures via Right Radial versus Left Radial Artery Approach: A Meta-Analysis. *Catheter Cardiovasc Interv.* 2016;*88*(7):1027–33.

13. Rashid M. Radial Artery Occlusion After Transradial Interventions: A Systematic Review and Meta-Analysis. *J Am Heart Assoc.* 2016;*5*(1):e002686.

14. Hahalis G. Radial Artery and Ulnar Artery Occlusions Following Coronary Procedures and the Impact of Anticoagulation: ARTEMIS (Radial and Ulnar Artery Occlusion Meta-Analysis) Systematic Review and Meta-Analysis. *J Am Heart Assoc.* 2017;*6*(8):e005430.

15. Sattur S. Transulnar Access for Coronary Angiography and Percutaneous Coronary Intervention. *J Invasive Cardiol.* 2014;*26*(8):404–8.

16. Kar S. Transulnar Cardiac Catheterization and Percutaneous Coronary Intervention: Techniques, Transradial Comparisons, Anatomical Considerations, and Comprehensive Literature Review. *Catheter Cardiovasc Interv.* 2017;*90*(7): 1126–34.

17. Kedev S. Safety and Feasibility of Transulnar Catheterization When Ipsilateral Radial Access Is Not Available. *Catheter Cardiovasc Interv.* 2014;*83*(1):E51–E60.

18. Rathore S. Impact of Length and Hydrophilic Coating of the Introducer Sheath on Radial Artery Spasm During Transradial Coronary Intervention: A Randomized Study. *J Am Coll Cardiol Intv.* 2010;*3*(5):475–83.

19. Jolly SS. Radial versus Femoral Access for Coronary Angiography and Intervention in Patients With Acute Coronary Syndromes (RIVAL): A Randomised, Parallel Group, Multicentre Trial. *The Lancet.* 2011;*377*(9775):1409–20.

20. Avdikos G. Radial Artery Occlusion After Transradial Coronary Catheterization. *Cardiovasc Diagn Ther.* 2017;*7*(3):305.

21. Schnyder G. Common Femoral Artery Anatomy Is Influenced by Demographics and Comorbidity: Implications for Cardiac and Peripheral Invasive Studies. *Catheter Cardiovasc Interv.* 2001;*53*(3):289–95.

22. Seto AH. Real-Time Ultrasound Guidance Facilitates Femoral Arterial Access and Reduces Vascular Complications: FAUST (Femoral Arterial Access With Ultrasound Trial). *J Am Coll Cardiol Intv.* 2010;*3*(7):751–58.

23. Ben-Dor I. Micropuncture Technique for Femoral Access Is Associated With Lower Vascular Complications Compared to Standard Needle. *Catheter Cardiovasc Interv.* 2021;*97*(7):1379–85.

24. Hildick-Smith DJ. Occasional-Operator Percutaneous Brachial Coronary Angiography: First, Do No Arm. *Catheter Cardiovasc Interv.* 2002;*57*(2):161–5.

25. Mele M. How Brachial Access Compares to Femoral Access for Invasive Cardiac Angiography When Radial Access Is Not Feasible: A Meta-Analysis. *J Vasc Access.* 2024;*25*(4):1063–8.
26. Karami M. Brachial Artery Access as a Novel Alternative for Impella 2.5 Insertion. *JACC Case Rep.* 2020;*2*(12):1884–7.

Radial-Specific Complication Management

12

Cara Hendry and Jonathan Hinton

12.1 INTRODUCTION

The use of the transradial approach (TRA) for coronary interventions has surpassed 90% of all percutaneous coronary intervention (PCI) cases in the United Kingdom, according to data reported nationally to NICOR [1]. The reasons for the selection of the TRA in comparison to transfemoral approach (TFA) have been discussed extensively in the first chapter of this text, but include patient preference, earlier ambulation, reduced vascular complication, bleeding risk, and mortality in patients receiving primary angioplasty in ST-segment elevation myocardial infarction (STEMI) [2, 3]. Major bleeding has been estimated to occur in 1% of TRA cases, and the major vascular complication rate is approximately 0.2% in a large, pooled analysis of the major randomised trials [4].

Complications involving the TRA nevertheless may occur and range from the development of small forearm haematoma to major bleeding or compartment syndrome requiring surgical treatment. It is therefore essential that operators and treating teams are aware of these so that patients may be properly informed for consent purposes and any complication may be managed in a safe and timely fashion to minimise any long-term or serious sequelae.

This chapter aims to outline the risk factors for and potential complications of the TRA and to highlight strategies for their prevention and treatment. Figure 12.1 describes a simplified approach to the management of these radial challenges.

DOI: 10.1201/9781003153627-12

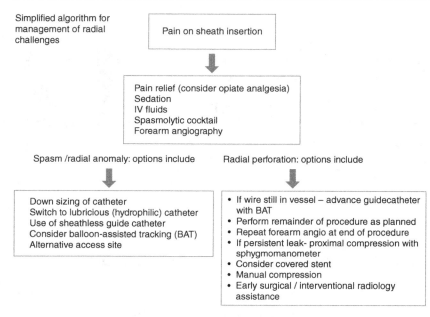

Simplified algorithm for management of radial challenges

Pain on sheath insertion

Pain relief (consider opiate analgesia)
Sedation
IV fluids
Spasmolytic cocktail
Forearm angiography

Spasm /radial anomaly: options include

Down sizing of catheter
Switch to lubricious (hydrophilic) catheter
Use of sheathless guide catheter
Consider balloon-assisted tracking (BAT)
Alternative access site

Radial perforation: options include

• If wire still in vessel – advance guidecatheter with BAT
• Perform remainder of procedure as planned
• Repeat forearm angio at end of procedure
• If persistent leak- proximal compression with sphygmomanometer
• Consider covered stent
• Manual compression
• Early surgical / interventional radiology assistance

FIGURE 12.1   Suggested algorithm for transradial challenges.

12.2 RISK FACTORS

12.2.1 Pre-procedural Risk Factors

There are a number of patient-related risk factors for access site complications. Identification of these facilitates the use of up-front strategies to prevent technical difficulty and potential complications. Patient-related risk factors for TRA complications include increased age, female gender, low body mass index, diabetes mellitus, South Asian ethnicity, and previous transradial procedures [5, 6]. Patients who are severely unwell at the time of the procedure (for example, those with advanced cardiogenic shock receiving high-dose vasoconstrictor therapy) and those with complex comorbidities (such as systemic vasculitic connective tissue disorders) are also at increased risk of complications. Anticipatory use of sedation, adequate hydration, consideration of ultrasound-guided access, and use of small calibre and hydrophilic sheaths (to reduce sheath-to-artery ratio) may facilitate a safe, comfortable, and efficient procedure. In addition, particularly in the elderly, the use of the left radial should be considered because tortuosity in the subclavian artery can present challenges to accessing the ascending aorta and manipulating catheters.

12.2.2 Procedural Risk Factors

Once the sheath has been successfully inserted, the presence of anatomical anomalies may affect the ability to advance catheters, resulting in pain and resistance upon catheter manipulation. This may cause and present in the same way as radial spasm (discussed in Section 12.3.1). Post-mortem studies indicate radial anomalies to be present in 4%–18% of the population [7–9]. It has been proposed that radial angiography be undertaken after sheath insertion as part of routine practice [10]. One potential downside to the use of routine radial angiography is that it can be uncomfortable, even with a 50:50 contrast/saline mix, and therefore could result in spasm. Anatomical variations affecting the radial artery are a strong determinant of technical failure of procedures utilising the TRA, and early identification of these allows for procedural planning to prevent complications from arising. One such example may be the presence of a radial loop, which has been shown to lead to procedural failure in up to 37% of patients [9]. Based on limited data, it is reasonable to switch from right to left radial access in the case of a radial loop because the frequency of bilateral loops is relatively low (14.2%) [11].

12.3 PROCEDURAL CHALLENGES AND COMPLICATIONS

12.3.1 Radial Spasm

Radial spasm may adversely affect patient experience during TRA procedures, causing significant pain and distress if not recognised and treated promptly. A systematic review of 19 studies (>7,000 patients) suggests that radial spasm is common, occurring in up to 15% of cases [12]. Predictors of spasm include multiple puncture attempts [13], the presence of radial anomalies, small vessel size, and pain on sheath insertion. Untreated, it may increase the risk of catheter entrapment [14] and avulsion of the radial artery [15], which are serious and avoidable complications. In practice, the most common effect of radial spasm is prolongation of the procedure, and in some instances, operators may cross over to an alternative access site.

Spasm may present to clinicians as resistance when trying to advance or manipulate catheters. It is important to recognise this early to prevent patient discomfort and rapidly worsening spasm. Measures taken to address this may include the administration of intravenous fluids, the use of analgesic and/or sedative drugs such as fentanyl or midazolam, and a spasmolytic cocktail of calcium channel blockers (e.g., verapamil or diltiazem 2.5–5 mg) and/or nitroglycerine 100–200 micrograms administered through the arterial sheath (in the absence of contraindications). In some institutions, these drugs are administered prophylactically on a routine basis after sheath insertion. With increased TRA experience and the widespread use of hydrophilic low-profile sheaths, in many centres, this has become less common practice, with spasmolytic cocktail and sedation reserved for cases when early symptoms of spasm are detected. In addition, balloon-assisted tracking (BAT) or catheter-assisted tracking (CAT) can help to deliver catheters in cases of spasm.

12.3.2 Vasovagal Reactions

Vasovagal reactions may occur in response to various stimuli, including that of radial artery cannulation and manipulation of catheters within the body. It may initially present with signs such as yawning, nausea, and sweating and can progress to a marked or relative drop in heart rate with a significant reduction in mean arterial pressure. This is often seen in younger patients, especially when they are more nervous and can be precipitated by the pain of radial artery spasm. Therefore, anti-anxiolytics, analgesics, and intravenous fluids should be used liberally, especially in younger patients. Maintaining hydration prior to procedures may be useful rather than keeping patients nil by mouth. Establishing an intravenous fluid infusion on all patients as soon as they are on the catheter lab table has the advantage of ensuring that IV access is available and working and allows the rapid administration of extra fluid to counter the effects of any vasovagal reactions.

During a vasovagal reaction in the catheter lab, the blood pressure will often not drop enough for patients to pass out, and increasing central volume with intravenous fluids may be all that is required to terminate the reaction. If patients remain hypotensive and bradycardic despite at least 500–1,000 ml of intravenous fluid, they can be given intravenous atropine (600 mcg boluses) or glycopyrronium (400 mcg boluses). The latter drug is less likely to cross the blood-brain barrier and is preferable in elderly patients as atropine can cause significant antimuscarinic side effects, in particular confusion, especially in older patients.

12.3.3 Radial Artery Perforation

Radial perforation leading to continued uncontrolled bleeding is rare [16]. Identification is essential to prevent the development of forearm haematoma, which has the potential to progress into compartment syndrome and ischaemia of the forearm. This complication should be suspected when there is significant forearm pain or difficulty advancing catheters, and angiography of the forearm vessels must be undertaken without delay. The use of glycoprotein IIb/IIIa inhibitors has been shown to be associated with an increased risk of haematoma, and as such, they should be used with caution [17]. Where perforation is confirmed by contrast extravasation, there are a number of options available. Tamponading by inserting a long sheath [18] or by inserting diagnostic or guide catheters will stop bleeding in most cases [19]. However, passing guiding catheters through the site of perforation may be very uncomfortable for patients, and the tip of the catheter may create a razor-wire effect, causing increasing radial spasm and pain. BAT, in which the proximal balloon tip, when inflated, creates a tapered edge, which is easier to advance, with guide catheter tamponade [20] provides an elegant solution, enabling the procedure to be completed through the initial access site, sealing the perforation. An alternative strategy is CAT, which has the advantage that it can be performed over a standard 0.035″ guidewire. This involves placing a 4 or 5 French long (>110 cm) diagnostic multipurpose or pigtail catheter within a 6F or 7F guide catheter to facilitate the passage to the aorta (Figures 12.2 and 12.3).

In cases where radial perforation has been identified, it is recommended that forearm angiography is undertaken at the end of the procedure to determine the need for further measures. Often, completing the procedure with a standard guide will result in a successful tamponade; however, if extravasation persists, using a longer sheath and/or external compression with an inflated sphygmomanometer cuff should reduce further bleeding. The size and position of any haematoma should be documented in the patient's case note, along with the presence of distal pulses, sensation, function, and capillary refill time of the affected hand, and the patient should be reviewed frequently.

12.3.4 Catheter Entrapment

This may occur due to severe spasm in small or aberrant anatomy and is associated with pain and failure to advance or remove a catheter. Often, simple measures such as analgesia and vasodilators, as described earlier, may help. Over-torquing a catheter may result in kinking and loss of arterial pressure trace. If recognised early and using X-ray screening, back along the path of the catheter, manoeuvres may be reversed to unkink the catheter. If the kink in the

Management of radial perforation: Balloon-assisted tracking technique

If guidewire present proximal to perforation	If no proximal guidewire in place

1.	Ensure adequate analgesia and sedation
2.	Pass 4 or 5F JR4 or MPA1 diagnostic catheter to ascending aorta
3.	Remove standard guidewire and pass workhorse coronary wire to ascending aorta
4.	Remove diagnostic catheter by hydroplaning (visualising wire tip under fluoroscopy)
5.	Insert guide catheter of choice (with angioplasty wire fixed by assistant) just proximal to sheath under fluoroscopic guidance
6.	Pass 15–20mm length 2mm compliant balloon(for 6F guidecatheter) on wire with half of balloon proximal to catheter and remainder within catheter
7.	Inform the team that the radial pressure will be lost during balloon inflation
8.	Inflate balloon to nominal pressure
9.	Gently advance the guide catheter under fluoroscopic guidance with the balloon inflated
10.	When catheter in ascending aorta deflate balloon and switch to standard 0.35in J tip wire.

If no proximal guidewire in place
- Ensure adequate analgesia and sedation
- Under fluoroscopy attempt to pass a coronary guidewire along the vessel proximal to the dissection
- Follow steps 3-10

FIGURE 12.2   Management of perforation.

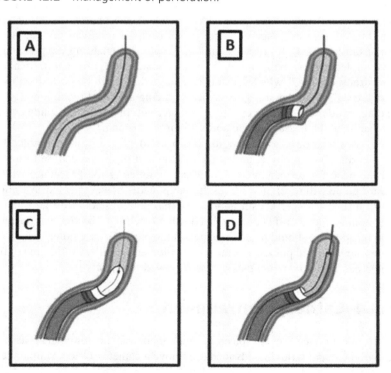

FIGURE 12.3   Use of BAT and CAT strategies to counter radial tortuosity or spasm. Panel A: Tortuous radial artery with standard 0.035″ wire across. Panel B: Stiff tip of guide catching in tortuosity. Panel C: BAT using a standard 0.014″ angioplasty wire and balloon. Panel D: CAT using standard 0.035″ wire with either 4 or 5 French long multipurpose catheter or 4 or 5F pigtail.

catheter cannot be untied, immobilising the catheter distal to the kink may be required and can be achieved either with external compression (with sphygmomanometer cuff or manual pressure at the brachial artery) or by snaring the distal end via another access site. If significant spasm continues to prevent removal of a catheter, the use of 3 mg intra-arterial boluses of papaverine has been reported to be effective. Alternatively, general anaesthesia may be required to allow the successful removal of a trapped catheter.

12.4 POST-PROCEDURAL COMPLICATIONS

12.4.1 Haematoma

Haematoma following TRA is commonly caused in one of two ways: bleeding from the puncture site (due to malposition of the haemostasis device or from multiple initial punctures) or from a more proximal perforation caused by inadvertent wire exit or trauma from passage of an over-sized guide catheter. As the radial and brachial arteries are both easily compressible, early recognition and action can avert more serious complications due to persistent bleeding. If repositioning of the haemostasis device or manual pressure over the puncture site fails to reduce the size of the haematoma, more proximal compression with a manual sphygmomanometer cuff, intermittently inflated to above systolic pressure for periods of five minutes should control any forearm bleeding.

Haematomas may be graded (Table 12.1) according to the EASY (Early Discharge After Transradial Stenting of Coronary Arteries) classification, ranging from grade I (<5 cm/superficial) to grade V (compartment syndrome with ischaemic threat to hand) [21]. The potential treatments were detailed earlier and should be instigated early to prevent continued bleeding and swelling in the forearm. Compartment syndrome should be suspected when there is forearm swelling associated with severe pain, especially with passive stretching of the fingers. For this reason, all members of the team involved in post-procedural care must be aware of the importance of close surveillance of patients with haematoma, with early escalation in the event of increased swelling in order to avoid the development of a compartment syndrome requiring surgical treatment.

Developing compartment syndrome is an emergency situation that requires immediate intervention. Most cases of compartment syndrome are related to limb fractures, and orthopaedic teams have experience and expertise in managing this limb-threatening complication by measuring pressures in the arm compartments and performing early decompressive surgery if indicated. They should be contacted as soon as a large haematoma is recognised.

TABLE 12.1   The EASY (Early Discharge After Transradial Stenting of Coronary Arteries) haematoma classification

GRADE	SIGNIFICANCE	SIZE (CM)	LOCATION
I	Non-significant	<5	Distal to elbow
II	Mild	5–10	Distal to elbow
III	Moderate	>10	Distal to elbow
IV	Severe	>10	Extending above elbow
V	Compartment syndrome with threat of hand ischaemia		Anywhere

12.4.2 Radial Artery Occlusion (RAO)

The development of RAO, although asymptomatic, is undesirable, as it may prevent future interventional procedures from being performed through the ipsilateral radial artery or its use for harvesting as a bypass graft conduit or for creation of AV fistula in renal failure should these procedures be required. The frequency of RAO after TRA is difficult to quantify, as preventative measures and diagnostic techniques vary widely. Furthermore, patients are unaware of its development. Meta-analyses suggest that the frequency varies widely (from <1% to 33%), depending on the timing of assessment [22]. The PROPHET II study data would suggest that with optimal technique and small sheath size, the RAO rates may be reduced to <3% [23]. Strategies to avoid RAO are similar to those adopted for prevention of radial artery spasm: limiting the number of punctures, using smaller sheath sizes, using hydrophilic low-profile sheaths, and considering the use of sheathless guide catheters. Anticoagulation is essential in avoidance of RAO; however, the optimal heparin dose is unclear, and many operators use 5,000 units of heparin, or 50 units/kg, as part of their standard protocol. Compression with patent haemostasis (discussed in Chapter 6) is a key component of prevention of RAO. Prior to discharge, all patients should be assessed using a reverse Barbeau test. If this suggests that RAO is present, then intervention with ipsilateral ulnar compression or a course of anticoagulant therapy will increase the rate of radial recanalisation.

12.4.3 Other Complications

Other complications which may arise as a result of TRA include pseudo-aneurysm formation, which is rare (<0.1%) but occurs more commonly in anti-coagulated patients and is often due to inadequate initial haemostasis at the puncture site. It presents as pulsatile swelling (which may or may not be painful) at the puncture site and is diagnosed by ultrasonography. Treatment depends on size and may include prolonged compression, thrombin injection, or surgical repair.

Arteriovenous fistula formation is exceedingly rare and should be suspected if there is an audible bruit or thrill over the artery on palpation. The shunt is often small and can be managed conservatively if asymptomatic.

Hand dysfunction has also been reported as pain or altered grip strength (<0.5%) [24, 25], as well as chronic regional pain syndrome, which is exceedingly rare. Early recognition should lead to a referral for active mobilisation and rehabilitation, as immobilisation will exacerbate the symptoms.

Other very rare but potentially serious complications include haemothorax or mediastinal haemorrhage [26]; these are caused by inadvertent wire exit of branches en route to the ascending aorta (such as the internal mammary or thyrocervical arteries), most commonly when using hydrophilic coated wires. Therefore, it is advised to use X-ray screening at all times to visualise passage of the tip of these hydrophilic wires while they are being advanced. Unexplained signs of progressive hypovolaemia should lead to urgent CT scanning and vascular intervention to control bleeding.

Critical hand ischaemia following TRA has often been described [27] in complex patients with significant pre-existing vascular disease, where RAO may have a more important impact. Additionally, distal embolisation may cause digital ischaemia, which may require alternative management with anticoagulation, as well as avoiding further invasive procedures that may lead to additional embolisation. Patients present with pallor and evident digital ischaemia. This is an urgent situation which may lead to amputation. The occurrence of hand ischaemia should be managed with multidisciplinary input from vascular surgeons and interventional radiologists. Options include anticoagulation, vasodilators, nerve block, thrombolysis, and vascular intervention.

12.5 CONCLUSIONS

Despite the potential complications which may arise as a result of TRA, it remains the access site of choice due to its benefits in terms of patient experience and superior patient safety profile in comparison to the TFA. Awareness of the potential risks which may arise is key, as early recognition and treatment can minimise these and potentially prevent the development of long-term sequelae.

REFERENCES

1. https://www.bcis.org.uk/audit-results/
2. Rao SV, Tremmel JA, Gilchrist IC, Shah PB, Gulati R, Shroff AR, Crisco V, Woody W, Zoghbi G, Duffy PL, et al. Society for Cardiovascular Angiography and Intervention's Transradial Working Group. Best Practices for Transradial Angiography and Intervention: A Consensus Statement From the Society for Cardiovascular Angiography and Intervention's Transradial Working Group. *Catheter Cardiovasc Interv.* 2014;*83*:228–36.
3. Dworeck C, Redfors B, Völz S, Haraldsson I, Angerås O, Råmunddal T, Ioanes D, Myredal A, Odenstedt J, Hirlekar G, Koul S, Fröbert O, Linder R, Venetsanos D, Hofmann R, Ulvenstam A, Petursson P, Sarno G, James S, Erlinge D, Omerovic E. Radial Artery Access Is Associated With Lower Mortality in Patients Undergoing Primary PCI: A Report From the SWEDEHEART Registry. *Eur Heart J Acute Cardiovasc Care.* 2020 Jun;*9*(4):323–32.
4. Ferrante G, Rao SV, Juni P, Da Costa BR, Reimers B, Condorelli G, Anzuni A, Jolly SS, Bertrand OF, Krucoff MW, et al. Radial versus Femoral Access for Coronary Interventions Across the Entire Spectrum of Patients With Coronary Artery Disease: A Meta-Analysis of Randomised Trials. *JACC Cardiovasc Intrev.* 2016;*9*:1419–34.
5. Abdelaal E, Molin P, Plourde G, et al. Successive Transradial Access for Coronary Procedures: Experience of Quebec Heart-Lung Institute. *Am Heart J.* 2013;*165*:325–31.
6. Kotowycz MA, Johnston KW, Ivanov J, et al. Predictors of Radial Artery Size in Patients Undergoing Cardiac Catheterization: Insights From the Good Radial Artery Size Prediction (GRASP) Study. *Can J Cardiol.* 2014;*30*:211.
7. Rodriguez-Niedenfuhr M, Vazquez T, Nearn L, et al. Variations of the Arterial Pattern in the Upper Limb Revisited: A Morphological and Statistical Study, With A Review of the Literature. *J Anat.* 2001;*199*(Pt 5):547–66.
8. McCormack LJ, Cauldwell EW, Anson BJ. Brachial and Antebrachial Arterial Patterns: A Study of 750 Extremities. *Surg Gynecol, Obstet.* 1953;*96*:43–54.
9. Barbeau GR Radial Loop and Extreme Vessel Tortuosity in the Trans-Radial Approach; Advantage of Hydrophilic-Coated Guidewires and Catheters. *Cather Cardiovasc Interv.* 2003;*59*:442–50.
10. Lo TS, Nolan J, Fountzopoulos E, et al. Radial Artery Anomaly and Its Influence on Transradial Coronary Procedural Outcome. *Heart* 2009;*95*:410–15.
11. Charalambous M, Soteriades E, Constantinides S, Christou C. Radial Artery Loops: Incidence and Management. *J Am Coll Cardiol.* 2014 Apr;*63*(12_ Supplement):A1806.
12. Kristić I, Lukenda J. Radial Artery Spasm During Transradial Coronary Procedures. *J Invasive Cardiol.* 2011;*23*:527–31.
13. Goldsmit A, Kiemeneij F, Gilchrist IC, Kantor P, Kedev S, Kwan T, Dharma S, Valdivieso L, Wenstemberg B, Patel T. Radial Artery Spasm Associated With Transradial Cardiovascular Procedures: Results From the RAS Registry. *Catheter Cardiovasc Interv.* 2014;*83*:E32–6.
14. Pancholy SB, Karuparthi PR, Gulati R. A Novel Nonpharmacologic Technique to Remove Entrapped Radial Sheath. *Catheter Cardiovasc Interv.* 2015;*85*:E35–8.

15. Dieter RS, Akef A, Wolff M. Eversion Endarterectomy Complicating Radial Artery Access for Left Heart Catheterization. *Catheter Cardiovasc Interv.* 2003 Apr;*58*(4):478–80.

16. Sanmartín M, Cuevas D, Goicolea J, Ruiz-Salmerón R, Gómez M, Argibay V. Complicaciones vasculares asociadas al acceso transradial para el cateterismo cardíaco [Vascular Complications Associated With Radial Artery Access for Cardiac Catheterization]. *Rev Esp Cardiol.* 2004 Jun;*57*(6):581–4.

17. Garg N, Umamaheswar KL, Kapoor A, Tewari S, Khanna R, Kumar S, Goel PK. Incidence and Predictors of Forearm Hematoma During the Transradial Approach for Percutaneous Coronary Interventions. *Indian Heart J.* 2019 Mar-Apr;*71*(2):136–42. doi: 10.1016/j.ihj.2019.04.014

18. Calviño-Santos RA, Vázquez-Rodríguez JM, Salgado-Fernández J, Vázquez-González N, Pérez-Fernández R, Vázquez-Rey E, et al. Management of Iatrogenic Radial Artery Perforation. *Catheter Cardiovasc Interv.* 2004;*61*:74–8.

19. Patel T, Shah S, Sanghavi K, Pancholy S. Management of Radial and Brachial Artery Perforations During Transradial Procedures—A Practical Approach. *J Invasive Cardiol.* 2009;*21*:544–47.

20. George S, Mamas M, Nolan J, Ratib K. Radial Artery Perforation Treated With Balloon Tracking and Guide Catheter Tamponade – A Case Series. *Cardiovasc Revasc Med.* 2016;*17*:480–6. doi: 10.1016/j.carrev.2016.06.005

21. Bertrand OF, Larose E, Rodés-Cabau J, Gleeton O, Taillon I, Roy L, Poirier P, Costerousse O, Larochellière RD. Incidence, Predictors, and Clinical Impact of Bleeding After Transradial Coronary Stenting and Maximal Antiplatelet Therapy. *Am Heart J.* 2009;*157*:164–9. doi: 10.1016/j.ahj.2008.09.010

22. Rashid M, Kwok CS, Pancholy S, Chugh S, Kedev SA, Bernat I, Ratib K, Large A, Fraser D, Nolan J, et al. Radial Artery Occlusion After Transradial Interventions: A Systematic Review and Meta-Analysis. *J Am Heart Assoc.* 2016;*5*:e002686. doi: 10.1161/JAHA.115.002686

23. Pancholy SB, Bernat I, Bertrand OF, Patel TM. Prevention of Radial Artery Occlusion After Transradial Catheterization: The PROPHET-II Randomized Trial. *JACC Cardiovasc Interv.* 2016;*9*:1992–9. doi: 10.1016/j.jcin.2016.07.020

24. Ul Haq MA, Rashid M, Kwok CS, Wong CW, Nolan J, Mamas MA. Hand Dysfunction After Transradial Artery Catheterization for Coronary Procedures. *World J Cardiol.* 2017;*9*:609–19. doi: 10.4330/wjc.v9.i7.609

25. Ayyaz Ul Haq M, Rashid M, Gilchrist IC, Bertrand O, Kwok CS, Wong CW, Mansour HM, Baghdaddy Y, Nolan J, Van Leeuwen MAH, et al. Incidence and Clinical Course of Limb Dysfunction Post Cardiac Catheterization – A Systematic Review. *Circ J.* 2018;*82*:2736–44.

26. Wang K, Wen L, Xie L, et al. Giant Thoracic Hematoma Post-Transradial Coronary Angiography: A Case Report and Review of the Literature. *BMC Cardiovasc Disord.* 2023;*23*:442. doi: 10.1186/s12872-023-03466-7

27. Bojakowski K, Zawadzki M, Mruk B, Andziak P, Walecki J. Critical Hand Ischemia After Radial Access for Coronary Angiography – Case Report. *Pol J Radiol.* 2017 Jan 12;*82*:19–23. doi: 10.12659/PJR.899334

Index

Note that page numbers in **bold** represent tables, while those in *italics* represent figures.